JUST THE FACTS

ECG Interpretation

JUST THE FACTS

ECG Interpretation

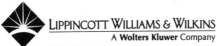

LIPPINCOTT WILLIAMS & WILKINS
A **Wolters Kluwer** Company

Philadelphia • Baltimore • New York • London
Buenos Aires • Hong Kong • Sydney • Tokyo

STAFF

Executive Publisher
Judith A. Schilling McCann,
RN, MSN

Editorial Director
William J. Kelly

Clinical Director
Joan M. Robinson, RN, MSN

Senior Art Director
Arlene Putterman

Editorial Project Manager
Ann E. Houska

Clinical Project Manager
Mary Perrong, RN, CRNP, MSN,
APRN,BC, CPAN

Editor
Catherine E. Harold

Clinical Editors
Karen A. Hamel, RN, BSN;
Pamela Kovach, RN, BSN

Copy Editors
Kimberly Bilotta (supervisor),
Tom DeZego

Designers
Linda Franklin (project
manager), Will Boehm (book
designer)

Digital Composition Services
Diane Paluba (manager),
Joyce Rossi Biletz,
Donna S. Morris

Manufacturing
Patricia K. Dorshaw (director),
Beth J. Welsh

Editorial Assistants
Megan L. Aldinger,
Tara L. Carter-Bell, Linda K. Ruhf

Indexer
Barbara Hodgson

JTFECG—D   N   O   S   A   J
06 05 04   10 9 8 7 6 5 4 3 2 1

**Library of Congress
Cataloging-in-Publication Data**

Just the facts : ECG interpretation.
    p. ; cm.
  Includes bibliographical references and index.
  1. Electrocardiography—Handbooks, manuals,
etc. 2. Cardiovascular system—Diseases—Nursing—Handbooks, manuals, etc. I. Lippincott
Williams & Wilkins. II. Title: ECG interpretation.
  [DNLM: 1. Electrocardiography—Handbooks.
2. Electrocardiography—Nurses' Instruction.
3. Arrhythmia—diagnosis—Handbooks. 4.
Arrhythmia—diagnosis—Nurses' Instruction. 5.
Heart Diseases—diagnosis—Handbooks. 6.
Heart Diseases—diagnosis—Nurses' Instruction.
WG 140 J96 2004]
RC683.5.E5J87 2004
616.1'207547—dc22
ISBN 1-58255-341-6 (alk. paper)   2004005312

Contents

Contributors and consultants

Linda S. Baas, RN, PhD, ACNP
Associate Professor and
   Director, Acute Care Graduate
   Program
University of Cincinnati College
   of Nursing

Nancy Bekken, RN, MS, CCRN
Staff Educator
Spectrum Health
Grand Rapids, Mich.

Deirdre Herr Byers, RN, BSN,
   CCRN
Staff Nurse, CCU
Southeast Georgia Regional
   Medical Center
Brunswick

Mary Lou Fisher, RN, BSN, MSN,
   CRNP, CCRN
Adult Nurse Practitioner
Johns Hopkins University
   Hospital
Baltimore

Dale Tomlinson Link, RN, MN,
   CNS
Clinical Care Coordinator,
   Cardiovascular Services
University of Alabama at
   Birmingham

Catherine Pence, RN, MSN, CCRN
Assistant Professor
Good Samaritan College of
   Nursing
Cincinnati

Janis Smith-Love, ARNP-C, MSN,
   CCRN, CEN
Cardiology Nurse Practitioner
Private Practice of David E.
   Perloff, MD, FACC, FACP
Fort Lauderdale, Fla.

Demetra C. Zalman, RN, BSN,
   CCRN
Staff Nurse
Hospital of the University of
   Pennsylvania
Philadelphia

Foreword

Most nurses and other health care professionals don't learn a lot about electrocardiography in school. But practitioners in virtually every clinical setting need at least a basic understanding of electrocardiography and its implications in practice.

Over the years, many students and clinicians have asked me to recommend a book that covers electrocardiogram (ECG) interpretation quickly and simply but with enough detail to build knowledge and confidence. Until now, I haven't had much to recommend because most ECG books are so complicated and impractical that even interested nurses lose heart.

That's why I'm delighted with *Just the Facts: ECG Interpretation*. Here's a book with an unusual combination of traits: It's both compact and comprehensive. The information is tightly targeted on essential facts and practical advice, all presented in a handy combination of bulleted lists and illustrations. This book was written with the clinician in mind. It includes not only the key information you need to interpret an ECG strip, but also the practical approach you need to respond appropriately in a clinical setting.

The first chapter, *Basic electrocardiography*, offers an introduction that covers leads, planes, types of ECG recordings and monitoring systems, electrode placement, waveform components, and an 8-step method for interpreting the ECG. This 8-step tool systematically simplifies rather than needlessly complicates the details of ECG interpretation.

Chapters 2 through 6 address the full spectrum of arrhythmia interpretation—including sinus node, atrial, junctional, and ventricular arrhythmias and atrioventricular blocks. For each arrhythmia, you'll find a concise description of key traits, an ECG strip, and a full review of causes, clinical significance, signs and symptoms, interventions, and management.

Chapters 7, 8, and 9 offer practical advice on detecting and responding to electrolyte effects, drug effects, and pacemaker and implantable cardioverter-defibrillator effects on the ECG. The final two chapters contain essential facts about 12-lead and advanced electrocardiography.

And there's more. Throughout the book, a special "Red flag" icon draws your attention to especially important information. Six helpful appendices are included: *Quick guide to cardiac arrhythmias* summarizes the details of 20 arrhythmias; *Cardiac drug overview* covers commonly used cardiac drugs; *Best monitoring leads* shows the most beneficial leads to monitor for the most challenging arrhythmias; *Depolarization-repolarization cycle* explains the five phases of this cardiac cycle; *Action potential curves* reviews the cellular changes that occur during the depolarization-repolarization cycle; and *Cardiac conduction system* reviews how electrical impulses affect heart function.

This clear, concise, and interesting new book is a wonderful reference for nurses, nurse practitioners, nursing students, and other health care professionals who need to understand electrocardiography from a clinician's viewpoint. With this book, any health care professional can achieve a rapid—and thorough—grasp of this sophisticated and increasingly important field.

Shu-Fen Wung, RN, PHD, ACNP
Associate Professor
University of Arizona
Tucson

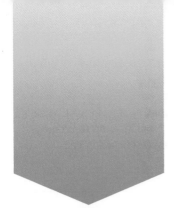

1

Basic electrocardiography

Electrocardiogram review

◆ Records the heart's electrical activity as waveforms that depict depolarization (contraction) and repolarization (relaxation).
◆ Aids in diagnosing and monitoring certain disorders:
  – Myocardial infarction.
  – Pericarditis.
◆ Allows identification of rhythm disturbances, conduction abnormalities, and electrolyte imbalances.

Leads

◆ Each lead provides a view of the heart's electrical activity between one positive and one negative pole.
◆ Each lead generates characteristic waveforms based on the direction electrical current is flowing.

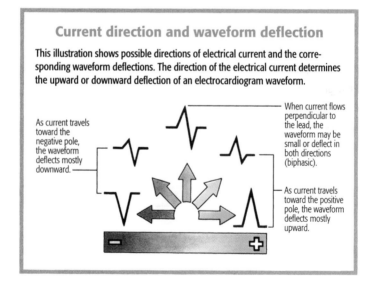

Current direction and waveform deflection

This illustration shows possible directions of electrical current and the corresponding waveform deflections. The direction of the electrical current determines the upward or downward deflection of an electrocardiogram waveform.

When current flows perpendicular to the lead, the waveform may be small or deflect in both directions (biphasic).

As current travels toward the negative pole, the waveform deflects mostly downward.

As current travels toward the positive pole, the waveform deflects mostly upward.

Planes

- Each plane is a cross-section of the heart that provides a different view of the heart's electrical activity.
- The six limb leads are viewed from the frontal plane.
- The six precordial leads are viewed from the horizontal plane.

12-lead ECG

- Information is recorded from 12 different views of the heart by electrodes on the patient's limbs and chest.
- Six limb leads (I, II, III, aV_R, aV_L, aV_F):
    – Provide information about the frontal plane of the heart.
    – May be bipolar and thus require a negative and positive electrode for monitoring (leads I, II, and III).
    – May be unipolar and thus need only a positive electrode (augmented leads aV_R, aV_L, aV_F).
- Six precordial leads (V_1, V_2, V_3, V_4, V_5, V_6):
    – Provide information about the horizontal plane of the heart.
    – Are unipolar (need only a positive electrode).
    – Allow calculation of the negative pole of the lead (in the center of the heart) by the electrocardiogram (ECG) monitor.

Single-lead or dual-lead ECG

◆ Monitor up to two different leads.
◆ Display heart rate.
◆ Commonly monitored leads:
   – I, II, and III.
   – MCL_1 (modified chest lead) and MCL_6 (similar to the unipolar leads V_1 and V_6 of the 12-lead ECG).

Dual-lead monitoring

Monitoring in two leads provides a more complete picture than monitoring in one. With simultaneous dual monitoring, you'll usually review the first lead – usually designated as the primary lead – for arrhythmias.

   A two-lead view helps detect ectopic beats or aberrant rhythms. Leads II and V_1 are the leads most commonly monitored simultaneously.

Lead II

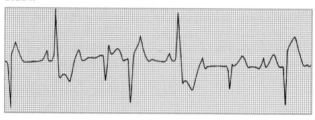

Lead V_1

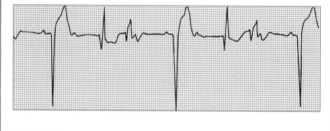

ECG monitoring systems

◆ May be hardwire or telemetry based on the patient's clinical status.
◆ Hardwire monitoring:
  – Provides direct connection between electrodes and cardiac monitor.
  – Permits continuous observation of one or more patients from more than one area of the unit.
  – Limits mobility because the patient is tethered to a monitor.
  – Provides a continuous cardiac rhythm display.
  – Transmits the ECG tracing to a console at the nurses' station.
  – Has alarms.
  – Has attachments that can track pulse oximetry, blood pressure, hemodynamic status, and other values.
◆ Telemetry monitoring:
  – Allows the patient to carry a small, battery-powered transmitter that sends electrical signals to another location for display on a monitor.
  – Useful for detecting arrhythmias during rest, sleep, exercise, and stressful situations.
  – Monitors only heart rate and rhythm.

Electrode placement

- ◆ Different for each lead. (See *Leadwire systems*, pages 8 and 9.)
- ◆ May highlight a particular part of the ECG complex or electrical events of a specific area of the heart.
- ◆ Leads II, V_1, and V_6 are common choices for continuous monitoring.
- ◆ May monitor in more than one lead.

Standard limb leads

- ◆ Lead I:
  - – Positive electrode on the left arm.
  - – Negative electrode on the right arm.
  - – Positive deflection.
  - – Helpful in monitoring atrial rhythms.
- ◆ Lead II:
  - – Positive electrode on the left leg.
  - – Negative electrode on the right arm.
  - – Positive, high-voltage deflection resulting in tall P, R, and T waves.
  - – Useful for P wave identification; detecting sinus node arrhythmia, atrial arrhythmia, and monitoring the inferior wall of the left ventricle.
- ◆ Lead III:
  - – Positive electrode on the left leg.
  - – Negative electrode on the left arm.
  - – Positive deflection.
  - – Useful in monitoring atrial rhythms and the inferior wall of the left ventricle.

Einthoven's triangle

The axes of the three bipolar limb leads (I, II, and III) form a triangle shape known as *Einthoven's triangle.* Because the electrodes for these leads are about equidistant from the heart, the triangle is equilateral.

The axis of lead I extends from shoulder to shoulder, with the right arm lead being the negative electrode and the left arm lead being the positive electrode. The axis of lead II runs from the negative right arm lead electrode to the positive left leg lead electrode. The axis of lead III extends from the negative left arm lead electrode to the positive left leg lead electrode.

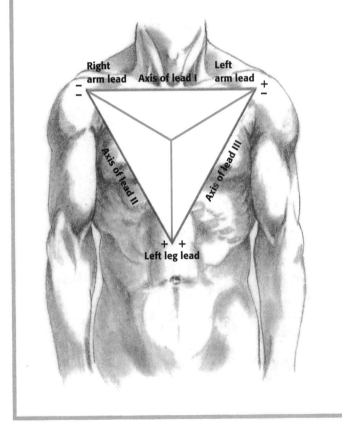

Leadwire systems

These illustrations show the correct electrode positions for some of the leads you'll use most often – the five-leadwire, three-leadwire, and telemetry systems. In the illustrations, RA stands for right arm, LA for left arm, RL for right leg, LL for left leg, C for chest, and G for ground.

Electrode positions

In the three- and five-leadwire systems, electrode positions for one lead may be identical to those for another lead. When that happens, change the lead selector switch to the setting that corresponds to the lead you want. In some cases, you'll need to reposition the electrodes.

Telemetry

In a telemetry monitoring system, you can create the same leads as the other systems with just two electrodes and a ground wire.

Five-leadwire system	Three-leadwire system	Telemetry system

Lead I

Lead II

Lead III

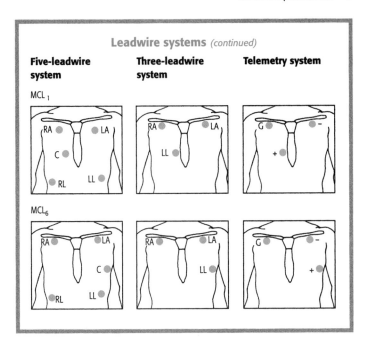

Leadwire systems *(continued)*

| **Five-leadwire system** | **Three-leadwire system** | **Telemetry system** |

Augmented unipolar leads

◆ Lead aV$_R$:
  – Positive electrode on the right arm.
  – Negative deflection.
◆ Lead aV$_L$:
  – Positive electrode on the left arm.
  – Usually a positive deflection.
◆ Lead aV$_F$:
  – Positive electrode on the left leg.
  – Positive deflection.
  – Inferior-wall changes shown well.

Precordial leads

◆ Six leads placed in sequence across the chest.
◆ Lead V_1 (corresponds to MCL_1):
  – Right side of the sternum at the fourth intercostal space.
  – Biphasic (positive and negative deflections).
  – P wave, QRS complex, and ST segment shown well.

Precordial views

These illustrations show the different views of the heart obtained from each precordial (chest) lead.

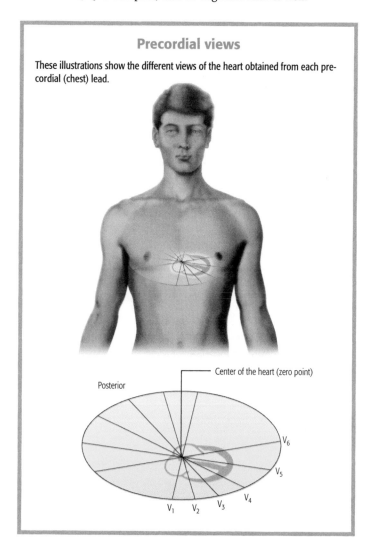

– Useful in monitoring ventricular arrhythmias, ST-segment changes, and P-wave changes.

– Useful in differentiating tachycardias (ventricular versus supraventricular) and bundle-branch blocks.

◆ Lead V_2:
– Left of the sternum at the fourth intercostal space.
– Negative deflection with a small amount of positive deflection.
– Used to detect ST-segment elevation.

◆ Lead V_3:
– Between V_2 and V_4 at the fifth intercostal space.
– Biphasic (positive and negative deflections).
– Used to detect ST-segment elevation.

◆ Lead V_4:
– Fifth intercostal space at the midclavicular line.
– Positive deflection.
– ST-segment and T-wave changes shown.

◆ Lead V_5:
– Fifth intercostal space at the anterior axillary line.
– Positive deflection.
– ST-segment and T-wave changes shown.

◆ Lead V_6 (equivalent to MCL_6):
– Fifth intercostal space at the midaxillary line.
– Positive deflection.

Modified chest leads

◆ MCL_1 (the lead equivalent of V_1 on the 12-lead ECG):
– Negative deflection.
– Used to assess QRS-complex arrhythmias, monitor premature ventricular beats and P-wave changes, distinguish different types of tachycardia (ventricular, supraventricular) and bundle-branch defects, and confirm pacemaker wire placement.

◆ MCL_6 (alternative to MCL_1):
– Same location as its equivalent, lead V_6.
– Monitors ventricular conduction changes.

ECG grid

◆ Waveforms produced by the heart's electrical current are recorded on electrocardiogram (ECG) graphing paper.

◆ The horizontal axis of the ECG strip represents time:
  – Each small block equals 0.04 second.
  – Five small blocks form a large block, which equals 0.2 second (0.04 second [one small block] multiplied by 5 [small blocks in a large block] = 0.2 second).
  – Five large blocks equal 1 second (5 × 0.2).
  – To measure or calculate heart rate, use a 6-second strip, which consists of 30 large blocks.

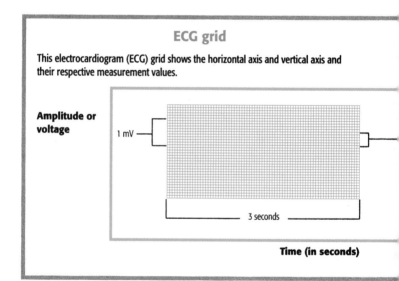

ECG grid

This electrocardiogram (ECG) grid shows the horizontal axis and vertical axis and their respective measurement values.

Amplitude or voltage

1 mV

3 seconds

Time (in seconds)

◆ The vertical axis of the ECG measures amplitude in millimeters (mm) or electrical voltage in millivolts (mV):
  – Each small block represents 1 mm or 0.1 mV.
  – Each large block represents 5 mm or 0.5 mV.
  – To determine the amplitude of a wave, segment, or interval, count the number of small blocks from the baseline to the highest or lowest point of the wave, segment, or interval on a standard 12-lead ECG.

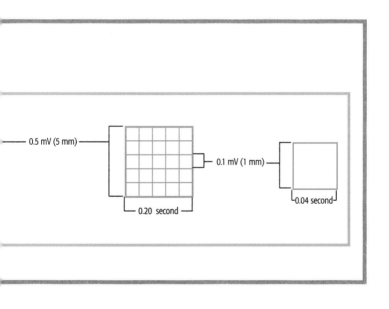

ECG complex

- ◆ Represents electrical events occurring in one cardiac cycle.
- ◆ Represents conduction of electrical impulses from the atria to the ventricles.
- ◆ Consists of five waveforms labeled with the letters P, Q, R, S, and T.
- ◆ Contains three elements (Q, R, and S) that form one unit, the QRS complex.

ECG waveform components

This illustration shows the components of a normal electrocardiogram (ECG) waveform.

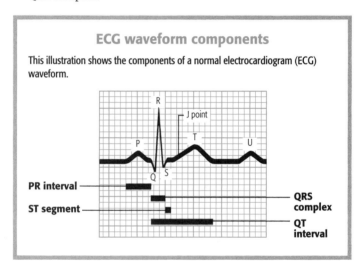

P wave

- ◆ Represents atrial depolarization or conduction of an electrical impulse through the atria.
- ◆ Location: Precedes the QRS complex.

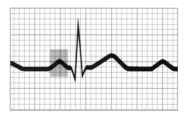

- Amplitude: 2 to 3 mm high.
- Duration: 0.06 to 0.12 second.
- Configuration: Usually rounded, upright.
- Deflection:
    - Positive or upright in leads I, II, aV_F, and V_2 to V_6.
    - Usually positive but may vary in leads III and aV_L.
    - Negative or inverted in lead aV_R.
    - Biphasic or variable in lead V_1.
- With normal deflection and configuration, assumption made that electrical impulses originated in the sinoatrial (SA) node.
- May represent atrial hypertrophy or enlargement if peaked, notched, or enlarged.
- May signify retrograde or reverse conduction from the atrioventricular (AV) junction toward the atria if inverted.
- Varying P waves indicate that the impulse may be coming from different sites.
- May signify conduction by a route other than the SA node if absent.
- May indicate complete heart block if P wave doesn't precede the QRS complex.

PR interval

- Tracks the atrial impulse from the atria through the AV node.
- Location: Start of the P wave to start of the QRS complex.

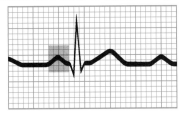

- Duration: 0.12 to 0.20 second:
    - Indicate that the impulse originated somewhere other than the SA node if less than 0.12 second.
    - Represent a conduction delay through the atria or AV junction if greater than 0.20 second.

QRS complex

♦ Represents depolarization of and impulse conduction through the ventricles, after which the ventricles contract and blood is ejected and pumped through the arteries, creating a pulse.

 RED FLAG *A QRS complex represents ventricular electrical activity but doesn't guarantee a mechanical contraction or a pulse. The contraction could be weak, as with premature ventricular contractions, or the contraction could be absent, as with pulseless electrical activity.*

♦ Location: Follows the PR interval.

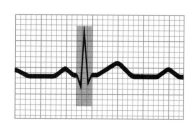

♦ Amplitude: 5 to 30 mm high, but differs for each lead used.
♦ Duration: 0.06 to 0.10 second, or half of the PR interval:
  – Measured from the start of the Q wave to the end of the S wave or from the start of the R wave if the Q wave is absent.
♦ Configuration:
  – Includes the Q wave (the first negative deflection, or deflection below the baseline, after the P wave), the R wave (the first positive deflection after the Q wave), and the S wave (the first negative deflection after the R wave).
  – May not display all three waves.
  – Will look different in each lead.
♦ Deflection:
  – Positive in leads I, II, III, aV_L, aV_F, and V_4 to V_6.
  – Negative in leads aV_R and V_1 to V_2.
  – Biphasic in lead V_3.

QRS waveform variety

The illustrations below show the various configurations of QRS complexes. When documenting the QRS complex, use uppercase letters to indicate a wave with a normal or high amplitude (greater than 5 mm) and lowercase letters to indicate one with a low amplitude (less than 5 mm).

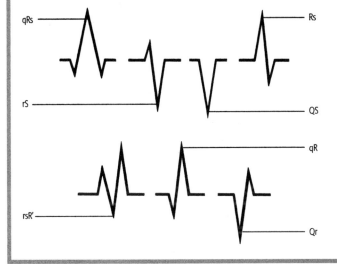

ST segment

◆ Represents the end of ventricular conduction or depolarization and the start of ventricular recovery or repolarization.
◆ J point: Marks the end of the QRS complex and the start of the ST segment.
◆ Location: From the S wave to the start of the T wave.

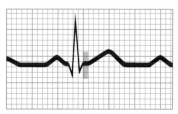

◆ Deflection:
  – Usually isoelectric (neither positive nor negative).
  – May vary from −0.5 to + 1 mm in some precordial leads.
◆ May become elevated or depressed.

Changes in the ST segment

Closely monitoring the ST segment on a patient's electrocardiogram can help you detect ischemia or injury before infarction develops.

ST-segment depression

An ST segment is considered depressed when it's 0.5 mm or more below the baseline. A depressed ST segment may indicate myocardial ischemia or digoxin use.

ST-segment elevation

An ST segment is considered elevated when it's 1 mm or more above the baseline. An elevated ST segment may indicate myocardial injury.

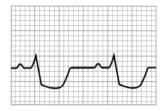

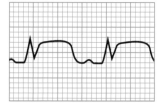

T wave

◆ Represents the relative refractory period of repolarization or ventricular recovery at peak.
◆ Location: Follows the ST segment.

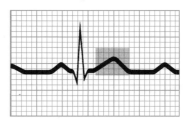

◆ Amplitude: 0.5 mm in leads I, II, and III and up to 10 mm in precordial leads.
◆ Configuration: Typically rounded and smooth.
◆ Deflection:
   – Usually positive or upright in leads I, II, aV_L, aV_F, and V_2 to V_6.
   – Inverted in lead aV_R.
   – Variable in leads III and V_1.
◆ If bumps in the T wave, may indicate hidden P wave.
◆ May indicate myocardial injury or electrolyte imbalances (hyperkalemia) if tall, peaked, or tented.
◆ May represent myocardial ischemia if inverted in leads I, II, aV_L, aV_F or V_2 through V_6.
◆ May mean pericarditis if heavily notched or pointed in an adult.

QT interval

◆ Measures the time needed for ventricular depolarization and repolarization.

◆ Location: The start of the QRS complex to the end of the T wave.

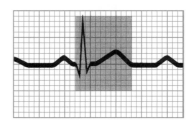

◆ Duration:
   – Varies with age, sex, and heart rate.
   – Lasts 0.36 to 0.44 second.
   – When the rhythm is regular, shouldn't be greater than half the distance between two consecutive R waves.

◆ If prolonged, indicates slowed ventricular repolarization, possibly from:
   – Effects of certain drugs such as Class I antiarrhythmics.
   – Prolonged QT syndrome (congenital conduction-system defect present in certain families).

◆ If shortened, may result from digoxin toxicity or electrolyte imbalances (such as hypercalcemia).

U wave

◆ Represents repolarization of the His-Purkinje system.
◆ May not appear on electrocardiogram.
◆ Location: Follows the T wave.

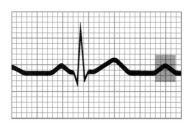

◆ Configuration: Typically upright, rounded.
◆ Deflection: Upright.
◆ If prominent, may be from hypercalcemia, hypokalemia, or digoxin toxicity.

8-step method of ECG evaluation

1. Determine rhythm

◆ Atrial rhythm:
  – Measure P-P intervals for several cycles. (See *Methods of measuring rhythm,* page 25.)
  – If consistently similar, atrial rhythm is regular.
  – If dissimilar, atrial rhythm is irregular.
◆ Ventricular rhythm:
  – Measure the intervals between two consecutive R waves in the QRS complexes.
  – If no R wave, use the Q wave or the S wave of consecutive QRS complexes.
  – If R-R intervals are consistently similar, ventricular rhythm is regular.
  – If dissimilar, ventricular rhythm is irregular.

2. Calculate rate

◆ Three methods to choose from: Times-10 method; 1,500 method; sequence method.
◆ Times-10 method:
  – Obtain a 6-second strip.
  – Count the number of P waves.
  – Multiply the number of P waves by 10 (ten 6-second strips equal 1 minute).
  – Calculate ventricular rate the same way using R waves.
◆ 1,500 method (because 1,500 small squares equal 1 minute):
  – Count the number of small squares between identical points on two consecutive P waves.
  – Divide the number by 1,500 to get the atrial rate.
  – Use the same method with two consecutive R waves to calculate the ventricular rate.
◆ Sequence method:
  – Find a P wave that peaks on a heavy lack line.
  – Assign these numbers to the next six heavy black lines: 300, 150, 100, 75, 60, and 50.
  – Find the next P wave peak.

– Estimate the atrial rate based on the number assigned to the nearest heavy black line.
– Estimate the ventricular rate the same way using the R wave.

3. Evaluate P wave
◆ Determine if a P wave is present for every QRS complex.
◆ Assess whether it has a normal configuration, size, and shape.

4. Determine PR interval duration
◆ Count small squares between the start of the P wave and the start of the QRS complex.
◆ Multiply the number of squares by 0.04 second.
◆ Determine if the duration is normal (0.12 to 0.20 second, or 3 to 5 small squares) and consistent.

5. Determine QRS complex duration
◆ Measure straight across from the beginning of the QRS complex to the end of the S wave (not just to the peak).
◆ Count the small squares between the beginning and end of the QRS complex.
◆ Multiply this number by 0.04 second.
◆ Determine if the duration is normal (0.06 to 0.10 second), all QRS complexes are the same size and shape, and a complex appears after every P wave.

6. Evaluate T wave
◆ Determine if T waves are present and have a normal shape, normal amplitude, and the same deflection as QRS complexes.
◆ Consider whether a P wave could be hidden in a T wave.

7. Determine QT interval duration
◆ Count the small squares between the beginning of the QRS complex and the end of the T wave (where the T wave returns to the baseline).
◆ Multiply this number by 0.04 second.
◆ Determine if the duration is normal (0.36 to 0.44 second).

8. Evaluate other components

◆ Make sure the waveform doesn't reflect problems with the monitor. (see *The look of monitor problems,* pages 26 to 29.)

◆ Note ectopic beats, aberrantly conducted beats, or other abnormalities.

◆ Check the ST segment for abnormalities.

◆ Look for a U wave.

◆ Classify the rhythm strip according to one or all of the following:

– Site of origin of the rhythm (sinus node, atria, atrioventricular node, or ventricles).

– Rate (normal [60 to 100 beats/minute], bradycardia [less than 60 beats/minute], tachycardia [more than 100 beats/minute]).

– Rhythm (normal or abnormal [flutter, fibrillation, heart block, escape rhythm, other arrhythmias]).

Methods of measuring rhythm

You can use either of the following methods to determine atrial or ventricular rhythm.

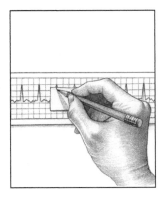

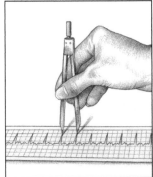

Paper-and-pencil method

Place the electrocardiogram (ECG) strip on a flat surface. Then position the straight edge of a piece of paper along the strip's baseline. Move the paper up slightly so the straight edge is near the peak of the R wave.

With a pencil, mark the paper at the R waves of two consecutive QRS complexes, as shown. This is the R-R interval. Next, move the paper across the strip lining up the two marks with succeeding R-R intervals. If the distance for each R-R interval is the same, the ventricular rhythm is regular. If the distance varies, the rhythm is irregular.

Use the same method to measure the distance between the P waves (the P-P interval) and determine whether the atrial rhythm is regular or irregular.

Caliper method

With the ECG on a flat surface, place one point of the calipers on the peak of the first R wave of two consecutive QRS complexes. Then adjust the caliper legs so the other point is on the peak of the next R wave, as shown. This distance is the R-R interval.

Next, pivot the first point of the calipers toward the third R wave and note whether it falls on the peak of that wave. Check succeeding R-R intervals in the same way. If they're all the same, the ventricular rhythm is regular. If they vary, the rhythm is irregular.

Using the same method, measure the P-P intervals to determine whether the atrial rhythm is regular or irregular.

The look of monitor problems

The following illustrations review commonly encountered monitor problems, how to identify them, possible causes, and possible interventions. Always assess the patient before troubleshooting the equipment.

Waveform	**Possible cause**
Artifact (waveform interference) 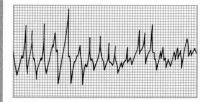	◆ Patient having seizures, chills, or anxiety
	◆ Dirty or corroded connections ◆ Improper electrode application
	◆ Short circuit in leadwires or cable
	◆ Electrical interference from other equipment in the room
	◆ Static electricity interference from inadequate room humidity
False-high-rate alarm 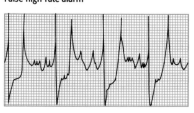	◆ Gain setting too high, particularly with MCL$_1$ setting
	◆ HIGH alarm set too low, or LOW alarm set too high
Weak signals 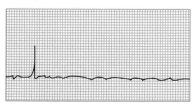	◆ Improper electrode application
	◆ QRS complex too small to register
	◆ Wire or cable failure

Interventions

◆ If the patient is having a seizure, notify the physician and intervene as needed.
◆ Keep the patient warm and encourage him to relax.

◆ Replace dirty or corroded wires.
◆ Check the electrodes and reapply them if needed. Clean the patient's skin well because skin oils and dead skin cells inhibit conduction.
◆ Check the electrode gel. If it's dry, apply new electrodes.

◆ Replace broken equipment.

◆ Make sure all electrical equipment is attached to a common ground. Check all three-prong plugs to make sure no prongs are loose. Notify the biomedical engineering department.

◆ Regulate room humidity to 40% if possible.

◆ Assess the patient for evidence of hyperkalemia.
◆ Reset gain.

◆ Set alarm limits according to the patient's heart rate.

◆ Reapply the electrodes.

◆ Reset gain so the height of the complex is more than 1 mV.
◆ Try monitoring the patient on another lead.

◆ Replace faulty wires or cables.

(continued)

The look of monitor problems *(continued)*

Waveform	Possible cause
Wandering baseline 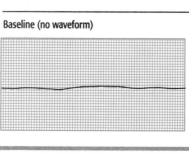	◆ Patient restless
	◆ Chest wall movement during respiration
	◆ Improper electrode application; electrode positioned over bone
Fuzzy baseline (electrical interference)	◆ Electrical interference from other equipment in the room
	◆ Improper grounding of the patient's bed
	◆ Electrode malfunction
Baseline (no waveform)	◆ Improper electrode placement (perpendicular to axis of heart)
	◆ Electrode disconnected ◆ Dry electrode gel
	◆ Wire or cable failure

Interventions

◆ Encourage the patient to relax.

◆ Make sure that tension on the cable isn't pulling the electrode away from the patient's body.

◆ Reposition improperly placed electrodes.

◆ Make sure all electrical equipment is attached to a common ground.
◆ Check all three-prong plugs to make sure no prongs are loose.

◆ Make sure the bed ground is attached to the room's common ground.

◆ Replace the electrodes.

◆ Reposition improperly placed electrodes.

◆ Check if electrodes are disconnected.
◆ Check electrode gel. If the gel is dry, apply new electrodes.

◆ Replace faulty wires or cables.

Normal sinus rhythm

- ◆ The norm against which all other rhythms are compared.
- ◆ Records an impulse that progresses to the ventricles through the normal conduction pathway.

Recognizing normal sinus rhythm

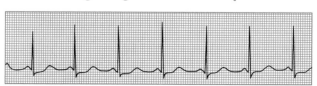

Electrocardiogram characteristics

- ◆ Rhythm
  - – Atrial rhythm regular.
  - – Ventricular rhythm regular.
- ◆ Rate
  - – 60 to 100 beats/minute.
  - – Sinoatrial node's normal firing rate.
- ◆ P wave
  - – Normal shape (round and smooth).
  - – Upright in lead II.
  - – All similar in size and shape.
  - – A P wave for every QRS complex.

- ◆ PR interval
  - – Within normal limits (0.12 to 0.20 second).
- ◆ QRS complex
  - – Within normal limits (0.06 to 0.10 second).
- ◆ T wave
  - – Normal shape.
  - – Upright and rounded in lead II.
- ◆ QT interval
  - – Within normal limits (0.36 to 0.44 second).
- ◆ Other
  - – No ectopic or aberrant beats.

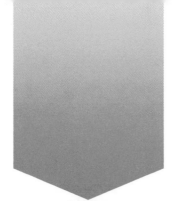

2

Sinus node arrhythmias

Sinus arrhythmia

- ◆ Rate:
  - – Within normal limits.
- ◆ Rhythm:
  - – Irregular.
  - – Corresponds to the respiratory cycle.
- ◆ Occurs as the heart's normal response to respiration.
- ◆ May be a normal finding in athletes, children, and older adults.
- ◆ Rarely occurs in infants.

Recognizing sinus arrhythmia

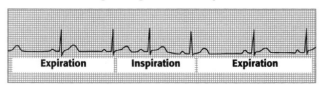

| Expiration | Inspiration | Expiration |

Electrocardiogram characteristics

- ◆ Rhythm
  - – Irregular.
  - – Corresponds to the respiratory cycle.
  - – P-P interval and R-R interval shorter during inspiration, longer during expiration.
  - – Difference between longest and shortest P-P interval exceeds 0.12 second.
- ◆ Rate
  - – Usually within normal limits (60 to 100 beats/minute).
  - – Varies with respiration.
  - – Increases during inspiration.
  - – Decreases during expiration.
- ◆ P wave
  - – Normal size.
  - – Normal configuration.

- ◆ PR interval
  - – May vary slightly.
  - – Within normal limits.
- ◆ QRS complex
  - – P wave before each QRS complex.
- ◆ T wave
  - – Normal size.
  - – Normal configuration.
- ◆ QT interval
  - – May vary slightly.
  - – Usually within normal limits.
- ◆ Other
  - – Phasic slowing and quickening.

Causes

◆ Inhibition of reflex vagal activity (tone).
◆ During inspiration:
  – Increased venous return.
  – Decreased vagal tone.
  – Increased heart rate.
◆ During expiration:
  – Decreased venous return.
  – Increased vagal tone.
  – Decreased heart rate.
◆ Other possible causes:
  – Heart disease.
  – Inferior-wall myocardial infarction.
  – Drugs (digoxin, morphine).
  – Increased intracranial pressure.

Clinical significance

◆ Usually insignificant.
◆ Usually produces no symptoms.
◆ May indicate sick sinus syndrome — a related but potentially more serious disorder — if marked variation in P-P intervals occurs in an older adult.

Signs and symptoms

◆ Peripheral pulse rate increases during inspiration and decreases during expiration.
◆ The arrhythmia may disappear when the patient's heart rate increases, as with exercise.
◆ If the arrhythmia results from an underlying condition, signs and symptoms of that condition may appear.
◆ A patient with marked sinus arrhythmia may develop dizziness or syncope.

Interventions

> RED FLAG *If sinus arrhythmia develops suddenly in a patient who's taking digoxin, notify the physician. The patient may have developed digoxin toxicity.*

- Treatment usually isn't needed if the patient is asymptomatic.
- If unrelated to respirations, treat underlying cause.
- If induced by drugs (morphine or another sedative), notify the physician, who will decide whether to continue giving the drug.

Sinus bradycardia

- ◆ Rate less than 60 beats/minute.
- ◆ Rhythm regular.
- ◆ Impulses originating in the sinus node.

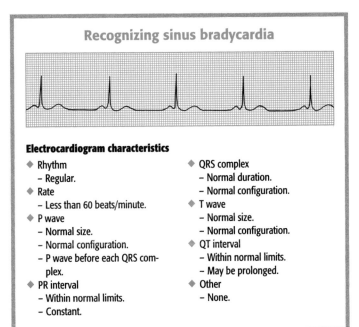

Recognizing sinus bradycardia

Electrocardiogram characteristics

- ◆ Rhythm
  - Regular.
- ◆ Rate
  - Less than 60 beats/minute.
- ◆ P wave
  - Normal size.
  - Normal configuration.
  - P wave before each QRS complex.
- ◆ PR interval
  - Within normal limits.
  - Constant.
- ◆ QRS complex
  - Normal duration.
  - Normal configuration.
- ◆ T wave
  - Normal size.
  - Normal configuration.
- ◆ QT interval
  - Within normal limits.
  - May be prolonged.
- ◆ Other
  - None.

Causes

- ◆ Noncardiac disorders:
  - Glaucoma.
  - Hyperkalemia.
  - Hypothermia.
  - Hypothyroidism.
  - Increased intracranial pressure.
- ◆ Conditions that increase vagal stimulation or decrease sympathetic stimulation:
  - Carotid sinus massage.
  - Deep relaxation.

- Sleep.
- Valsalva's maneuver.
- Vomiting.
◆ Cardiac diseases:
- Cardiomyopathy.
- Heart block.
- Inferior-wall myocardial infarction.
- Myocardial ischemia.
- Myocarditis.
- Sinoatrial node disease.
◆ Drugs:
- Antiarrhythmics (amiodarone, propafenone, quinidine, sotalol).
- Beta blockers.
- Calcium channel blockers.
- Digoxin.
- Lithium.

Clinical significance

◆ Significance depends on how low the rate is and whether the patient has symptoms.

 RED FLAG *If the patient has symptoms, prompt attention is critical. The heart of a patient with underlying cardiac disease may not be able to increase stroke volume to compensate for a decrease in rate. The resulting decline in cardiac output produces such signs and symptoms as hypotension and dizziness. Notify the physician immediately.*

◆ Sinus bradycardia may predispose some patients to more serious arrhythmias, such as ventricular tachycardia or ventricular fibrillation.

Signs and symptoms

◆ Pulse rate less than 60 beats/minute.
◆ Rhythm regular.
◆ No symptoms if the patient is able to compensate for the decreased cardiac output.
◆ If unable to compensate, cardiac output declines and symptoms develop:
  – Altered mental status.
  – Blurred vision.
  – Chest pain.
  – Cool, clammy skin.
  – Crackles.
  – Dizziness.
  – Dyspnea.
  – Hypotension.
  – S_3 heart sound, indicating heart failure.
  – Syncope.
◆ Bradycardia-induced syncope may occur and is known as a *Stokes-Adams attack.*

Interventions

◆ Usually, no treatment is needed if the patient has stable vital signs and no symptoms.
◆ Assess the heart rhythm and progression and duration of the bradycardia.
◆ Evaluate the patient's tolerance for the rhythm at rest and with activity.
◆ Review the patient's drugs.
◆ If the patient has symptoms of reduced cardiac output, identify and correct the underlying cause, if possible, and take steps to determine the proper treatment using a bradycardia algorithm. (See *Bradycardia algorithm,* pages 38 and 39.)
◆ Prepare patient for treatments as needed, such as drug administration (atropine, dopamine, epinephrine); transvenous or transcutaneous pacing; or permanent pacemaker insertion for a chronic, symptomatic condition.

Bradycardia algorithm

A patient with a bradycardic rhythm may either show few symptoms or symptoms of decreased cardiac output. If the patient does have decreased cardiac output, determine the cause and start appropriate treatments.

Bradycardia

- ◆ Slow (absolute bradycardia is less than 60 beats/minute) or
- ◆ Relatively slow (rate less than expected based on underlying condition or cause).

Primary ABCD* survey

- ◆ Assess ABCs.
- ◆ Secure airway noninvasively.
- ◆ Keep monitor or defibrillator available.

Secondary ABCD survey

- ◆ Assess secondary ABCs and need for invasive airway management.
- ◆ Initiate oxygen, I.V. access, monitor fluids.
- ◆ Monitor vital signs (especially blood pressure) and pulse oximetry.
- ◆ Obtain and review 12-lead electrocardiogram.
- ◆ Obtain and review portable chest X-ray.
- ◆ Obtain problem-focused history.
- ◆ Obtain problem-focused physical examination.
- ◆ Consider causes (differential diagnoses).

* Airway, breathing, circulation, defibrillation.

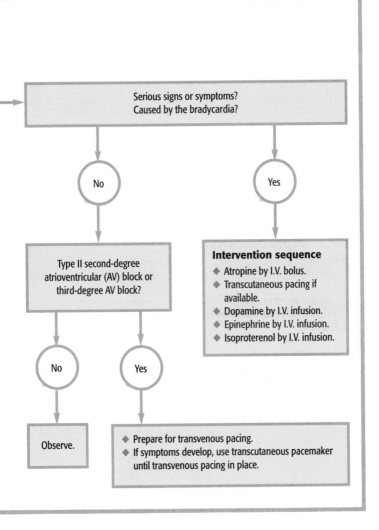

Sinus tachycardia

- ◆ Accelerated sinoatrial node firing.
- ◆ Sinus rate above 100 beats/minute in an adult.
- ◆ Rarely above 180 beats/minute except during strenuous exercise (maximum rate declining with age).

Recognizing sinus tachycardia

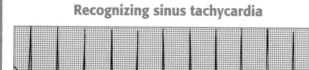

Electrocardiogram characteristics

- ◆ Rhythm
  - Regular.
- ◆ Rate
  - More than 100 beats/minute.
  - Usually 100 to 160 beats/minute.
- ◆ P wave
  - Normal size.
  - Normal configuration.
  - May increase in amplitude.
  - Precedes each QRS complex.
  - As heart rate increases, may be superimposed on preceding T wave and difficult to identify.

- ◆ PR interval
  - Within normal limits.
  - Constant.
- ◆ QRS complex
  - Normal duration.
  - Normal configuration.
- ◆ T wave
  - Normal size.
  - Normal configuration.
- ◆ QT interval
  - Within normal limits.
  - Commonly shortened.
- ◆ Other
  - None.

Causes

- ◆ May be a normal response:
  - – Exercise.
  - – Fever.
  - – Pain.
  - – Stress.
  - – Strong emotions (fear, anxiety).
- ◆ Cardiac conditions:
  - – Cardiogenic shock.
  - – Heart failure.
  - – Pericarditis.
- ◆ Other conditions
  - – Anemia.
  - – Hemorrhage.
  - – Hyperthyroidism.
  - – Hypovolemia.
  - – Pulmonary embolism.
  - – Respiratory distress.
  - – Sepsis.
- ◆ Drugs:
  - – Aminophylline.
  - – Amphetamines.
  - – Atropine.
  - – Dobutamine.
  - – Dopamine.
  - – Epinephrine.
  - – Isoproterenol.
- ◆ Lifestyle choices:
  - – Alcohol.
  - – Caffeine.
  - – Nicotine.

Clinical significance

- ◆ Depends on the underlying cause.
- ◆ None if results from exercise or strong emotions.
- ◆ May resolve spontaneously when condition (hypovolemia, hemorrhage, pain) resolves.
- ◆ May be serious if persistent, especially if it occurs with acute myocardial infarction.

Signs and symptoms

◆ Peripheral pulse rate above 100 beats/minute.
◆ Rhythm regular.
◆ Usually no symptoms.
◆ If cardiac output falls and compensatory mechanisms fail:
  – Anxiety.
  – Blurred vision.
  – Chest pain.
  – Hypotension.
  – Nervousness.
  – Palpitations.
  – Syncope.
◆ If heart failure develops:
  – Crackles.
  – S_3 heart sound.
  – Jugular vein distention.

 ## Interventions

◆ No treatment is needed if the patient is asymptomatic.
◆ Correct the underlying cause.
◆ If the patient has cardiac ischemia, give drugs to slow the heart rate:
  – Beta blockers (propranolol and atenolol).
  – Calcium channel blockers (verapamil and diltiazem).
◆ Ask the patient about use of tachycardia-triggering drugs and substances, and advise abstinence.

 RED FLAG *Notify the physician promptly if sinus tachycardia arises suddenly after a myocardial infarction. It may signal extension of the infarct.*

◆ Provide a calm environment, and help the patient with relaxation techniques.
◆ Help reduce the patient's fear and anxiety.

Sinus arrest

◆ Normal sinus rhythm with occasional, prolonged failure of sinoatrial (SA) node to initiate an impulse.
◆ Episodic failure in automaticity or impulse formation of the SA node and lack of atrial stimulation.
◆ PQRST complex or complexes missing.

Recognizing sinus arrest

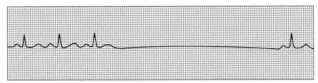

Electrocardiogram characteristics

◆ Rhythm
  – Regular except during arrest (irregular as result of missing complexes).
◆ Rate
  – Usually within normal limits (60 to 100 beats/minute) before arrest.
  – Length or frequency of pause may result in bradycardia.
◆ P wave
  – Periodically absent, with entire PQRST complexes missing.
  – When present, normal size and configuration.
  – Precedes each QRS complex.
◆ PR interval
  – Within normal limits when a P wave is present.
  – Constant when a P wave is present.

◆ QRS complex
  – Normal duration.
  – Normal configuration.
  – Absent during arrest.
◆ T wave
  – Normal size.
  – Normal configuration.
  – Absent during arrest.
◆ QT interval
  – Within normal limits.
  – Absent during arrest.
◆ Other
  – The pause with sinus arrest isn't equal to a multiple of the previous P-P intervals. Junctional escape beats may occur at end of pause.

Causes

◆ Acute infection.
◆ Sick sinus syndrome.
◆ Increased vagal tone.
◆ Sinus node disease.
◆ Cardioactive drugs:
  – Amiodarone.
  – Beta blockers (bisoprolol, metoprolol, propranolol).
  – Calcium channel blockers (diltiazem, verapamil).
  – Digoxin.
  – Quinidine.
  – Procainamide.
  – Salicylate toxicity.
◆ Cardiac disorders:
  – Acute inferior-wall myocardial infarction.
  – Acute myocarditis.
  – Cardiomyopathy.
  – Coronary artery disease.
  – Hypertensive heart disease.

Clinical significance

◆ Commonly, no symptoms.
◆ Syncope or near-syncopal episodes.
◆ During a prolonged pause, risk of falling or injury (such as a car accident if driving at the time).
◆ Risk of other arrhythmias from extremely slow rates.

Signs and symptoms

◆ Pulse and heart sounds absent during arrest.
◆ No symptoms with short pauses.
◆ Evidence of decreased cardiac output with recurrent or pro-longed pauses: low blood pressure; altered mental status; cool, clammy skin; syncope or near-syncope; dizziness; blurred vision.

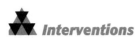
Interventions

♦ No treatment is needed if the patient is asymptomatic.
♦ If the patient has symptoms, follow the guidelines for responding to symptomatic bradycardia. (See *Bradycardia algorithm,* pages 38 and 39.)
♦ As needed, discontinue drugs that affect SA node discharge or conduction:
  – Beta blockers.
  – Calcium channel blockers.
  – Digoxin.

Sinoatrial exit block

◆ Regular discharges of sinoatrial (SA) node.
◆ Delayed or blocked SA node impulses with long sinus pauses.
◆ Pause of indefinite length ending with sinus rhythm.
◆ Possible lack of atrial activity.

Recognizing sinoatrial exit block

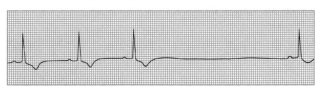

Electrocardiogram characteristics

◆ Rhythm
  – Regular except during pause (irregular as result of pause).
  – Absent during sinus arrest.
◆ Rate
  – Usually within normal limits (60 to 100 beats/minute) before pause.
  – Length or frequency of pause may result in bradycardia.
◆ P wave
  – Periodically absent, with entire PQRST complex missing.
  – When present, normal size and configuration.
  – Precedes each QRS complex.
◆ PR interval
  – Within normal limits.
  – Constant when a P wave is present.

◆ QRS complex
  – Normal duration.
  – Normal configuration.
  – Absent during a pause.
◆ T wave
  – Normal size.
  – Normal configuration.
  – Absent during a pause.
◆ QT interval
  – Within normal limits.
  – Absent during a pause.
◆ Other
  – The length of the pause may be a multiple of the underlying P-P interval.

Causes

◆ Acute infection.
◆ Sick sinus syndrome.
◆ Sinus node disease.
◆ Increased vagal tone.
◆ Cardioactive drugs:
  – Amiodarone.
  – Beta blockers (bisoprolol, metoprolol, propranolol).
  – Calcium channel blockers (diltiazem, verapamil).
  – Digoxin.
  – Quinidine.
  – Procainamide.
  – Salicylate toxicity.
◆ Cardiac disorders:
  – Acute inferior-wall myocardial infarction.
  – Acute myocarditis.
  – Cardiomyopathy.
  – Coronary artery disease.
  – Hypertensive heart disease.

Clinical significance

◆ Commonly, no symptoms.
◆ Syncope or near-syncope.
◆ During a prolonged pause, risk of falling or injury (such as a car accident if driving at the time).
◆ Risk of other arrhythmias from extremely slow rates.

Signs and symptoms

◆ Pulse and heart sounds absent during SA exit block.
◆ No symptoms with short pauses.
◆ Evidence of decreased cardiac output with recurrent or prolonged pauses:
  – Altered mental status.
  – Blurred vision.
  – Cool, clammy skin.
  – Dizziness.
  – Low blood pressure.
  – Syncope or near-syncope.

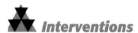

Interventions

◆ No treatment is needed if the patient has no symptoms.
◆ If the patient has symptoms, follow the guidelines for responding to symptomatic bradycardia. (See *Bradycardia algorithm,* pages 38 and 39.)
◆ As needed, discontinue drugs that affect SA node discharge or conduction:
 – Beta blockers.
 – Calcium channel blockers.
 – Digoxin.

Sick sinus syndrome

◆ Also known as *sinotrial (SA) syndrome, sinus nodal dysfunction,* and *Stokes-Adams syndrome.*
◆ Includes many SA node arrhythmias.

Recognizing sick sinus syndrome

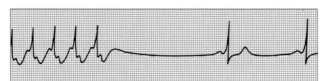

Electrocardiogram characteristics

◆ Rhythm
  – Irregular.
  – Sinus pauses.
  – Abrupt rate changes.
◆ Rate
  – Fast, slow, or alternating.
  – Interrupted by a long sinus pause.
◆ P wave
  – Varies with rhythm changes.
  – May be normal size and configuration.
  – May be absent.
  – Usually precedes each QRS complex.

◆ PR interval
  – Usually within normal limits.
  – Varies with rhythm changes.
◆ QRS complex
  – Duration within normal limits.
  – Varies with rhythm changes.
  – Normal configuration.
◆ T wave
  – Normal size.
  – Normal configuration.
◆ QT interval
  – Usually within normal limits.
  – Varies with rhythm changes.
◆ Other
  – Usually more than one arrhythmia on a 6-second strip.

Causes

◆ Conditions that affect the atrial wall around the SA node by causing inflammation or degeneration of atrial tissue, which may lead to exit blocks.
◆ Conditions leading to fibrosis of the SA node:
  – Advanced age.
  – Atherosclerotic heart disease.
  – Cardiomyopathy.
  – Hypertension.
◆ Trauma to the SA node:
  – Open-heart surgery, especially valve surgery.
  – Pericarditis.
  – Rheumatic heart disease.
◆ Autonomic disturbances affecting autonomic innervation:
  – Degeneration of autonomic system.
  – Hypervagotonia.
◆ Cardioactive drugs:
  – Beta blockers.
  – Calcium channel blockers.
  – Digoxin.

Clinical significance

◆ Depends on the patient's age and other diseases.
◆ Worse prognosis with atrial fibrillation because of the increased risk of thromboembolic complications.

Signs and symptoms

◆ Fast, slow, or normal pulse rate.
◆ Regular or irregular rhythm.
◆ No increase in heart rate with exertion.
◆ Episodes of tachy-brady syndrome, atrial flutter, atrial fibrillation, SA block, sinus arrest.
◆ If underlying cardiomyopathy:
  – Dilated and displaced left ventricular apical impulse.
  – Possible crackles.
  – S_3 heart sound.

◆ If thromboembolism:
- Acute pain.
- Blurred vision.
- Chest pain.
- Dyspnea.
- Fatigue.
- Hypotension.
- Neurologic changes (confusion, vision disturbances, weakness).
- Syncope (Stokes-Adams attacks).
- Tachycardia.
- Tachypnea.

Interventions

◆ No treatment is needed if the patient is asymptomatic.
◆ If symptoms develop, alleviate them and correct the underlying cause.
◆ If the patient has symptoms, follow the guidelines for responding to symptomatic bradycardia. (See *Bradycardia algorithm,* pages 38 and 39.)
◆ Prepare the patient for a temporary pacemaker.
◆ If arrhythmia results from a chronic disorder, treatment may consist of digoxin, a beta blocker, or radio-frequency ablation. A permanent pacemaker may be inserted to maintain heart rate and ensure adequate cardiac output.
◆ Administer anticoagulant for atrial fibrillation.
◆ Monitor the patient after starting beta blockers, calcium channel blockers, or other antiarrhythmics.

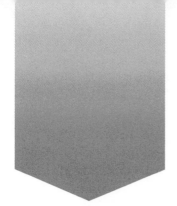

3

Atrial arrhythmias

Premature atrial contractions

◆ Origination:
  – In the atria.
  – Outside the sinoatrial (SA) node.
  – From a single ectopic focus or multiple atrial foci that supersede the SA node as pacemaker for one or more beats.

Recognizing premature atrial contractions

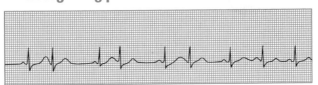

ECG characteristics

◆ Rhythm
  – Atrial: Irregular.
  – Ventricular: Irregular.
  – Underlying: May be regular.
◆ Rate
  – Atrial and ventricular: Vary with underlying rhythm.
◆ P wave
  – Premature.
  – Abnormal configuration compared to a sinus P wave.
  – If varying configurations, multiple ectopic sites.
  – May be hidden in preceding T wave.
◆ PR interval
  – Usually within normal limits.
  – May be shortened or slightly prolonged for the ectopic beat, depending on the origin of ectopic focus.

◆ QRS complex
  – Conducted: Duration and configuration usually normal.
  – Nonconducted: No QRS complex follows premature atrial contraction (PAC).
◆ T wave
  – Usually normal.
  – May be distorted if P wave is hidden in T wave.
◆ QT interval
  – Usually within normal limits.
◆ Other
  – May be a single beat.
  – May be bigeminal (every other beat premature).
  – May be trigeminal (every third beat premature).
  – May be quadrigeminal (every fourth beat premature).
  – May occur in couplets (pairs).
  – Three or more PACs in a row: atrial tachycardia.

◆ May be conducted or nonconducted (blocked) through AV node and heart depending on status of the AV node and intraventricular conduction system.
◆ Conducted premature atrial contractions (PACs):
  – Ventricular conduction usually normal.
◆ Nonconducted PACs:
  – Not followed by QRS complex.
  – May be difficult to distinguish from SA block.

Distinguishing nonconducted premature atrial contractions from sinoatrial block

To differentiate between nonconducted premature atrial contractions (PACs) and sinoatrial (SA) block, check the following:

◆ Whenever you see a pause in a rhythm, look carefully for a nonconducted P wave, which may occur before, during, or just after the T wave that precedes the pause.
◆ Compare the T wave that precedes the pause with other T waves in the rhythm strip. Look for distortion in its slopes or a difference in its height or shape. These clues show you where a nonconducted P wave may be hidden.

◆ If you find a P wave in the pause, check to see whether it's premature or it occurs earlier than subsequent sinus P waves. If it's premature (see the shaded area in the top rhythm strip), you can be sure it's a nonconducted PAC.
◆ If there's no P wave in the pause or T wave (see the shaded area in the bottom rhythm strip), then the rhythm is SA block.

Nonconducted PAC

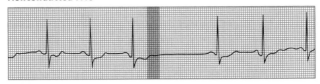

SA block

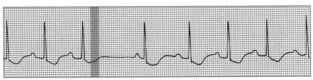

Causes

◆ Usually enhanced automaticity in atrial tissue.
◆ Trigger factors:
  – Alcohol.
  – Anxiety.
  – Cigarettes.
  – Fatigue.
  – Fever.
  – Infectious disease.
◆ Other causes:
  – Acute respiratory failure.
  – Chronic obstructive pulmonary disease.
  – Coronary heart disease.
  – Digoxin toxicity.
  – Drugs that prolong absolute refractory period of SA node, such as quinidine and procainamide.
  – Electrolyte imbalance.
  – Endogenous catecholamine release from pain or anxiety.
  – Hyperthyroidism.
  – Hypoxia.
  – Valvular heart disease.

Clinical significance

◆ Rarely dangerous if patient has no heart disease.
◆ Typically no symptoms; may go unrecognized for years.
◆ May lead to more serious arrhythmias, such as atrial fibrillation or flutter, if the patient has heart disease.

 RED FLAG *In a patient with acute myocardial infarction, PACs may be an early sign of heart failure or electrolyte imbalance.*

Signs and symptoms

◆ Pulse rhythm and rate that reflects underlying rhythm.
◆ Irregular peripheral or apical pulse rhythm when PACs occur.
◆ Sensation of palpitations, skipped beats, or fluttering.
◆ Evidence of decreased cardiac output, such as hypotension and syncope, if patient has heart disease.

 Interventions

◆ Usually, no treatment is needed if the patient has no symptoms.
◆ If the patient has symptoms, treatment may focus on eliminating or controlling the trigger factor, such as caffeine or alcohol consumption.
◆ Frequent PACs may be treated with drugs that prolong the atrial refractory period, such as beta blockers and calcium channel blockers.
◆ Tailor patient teaching to help the patient do the following:
  – Correct or avoid underlying causes, such as caffeine use.
  – Learn stress reduction techniques to lessen anxiety.
◆ If the patient has ischemic or valvular heart disease, watch for evidence of heart failure, electrolyte imbalance, and more severe atrial arrhythmias.

Atrial tachycardia

- A supraventricular tachycardia (impulses originate above the ventricles).
- Atrial rate: 150 to 250 beats/minute.
- Three forms discussed here:
  - Atrial tachycardia with block.
  - Multifocal atrial tachycardia (MAT, or chaotic atrial rhythm).
  - Paroxysmal atrial tachycardia (PAT), a transient event that starts and stops suddenly.

Recognizing atrial tachycardia

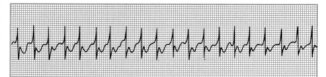

ECG characteristics

- Rhythm
  - Atrial: Usually regular.
  - Ventricular: Regular or irregular depending on atrioventricular (AV) conduction ratio and type of atrial tachycardia.
- Rate
  - Atrial: Three or more consecutive ectopic atrial beats at 150 to 250 beats/minute, rarely exceeding 250 beats/minute.
  - Ventricular: Depends on AV conduction ratio.
- P wave
  - May deviate from normal appearance.
  - May be hidden in preceding T wave.
  - If visible, usually upright and preceding each QRS complex.

- PR interval
  - May be unmeasurable if P wave can't be distinguished from preceding T wave.
- QRS complex
  - Duration and configuration usually normal.
  - May be abnormal if impulses conducted abnormally through ventricles.
- T wave
  - Usually visible.
  - May be distorted by P wave.
  - May be inverted if ischemia present.
- QT interval
  - Usually within normal limits.
  - May be shorter because of rapid rate.
- Other
  - May be difficult to differentiate atrial tachycardia with block from sinus arrhythmia with U waves.

Types of atrial tachycardia

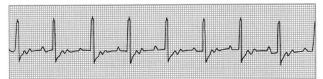

ECG characteristics of atrial tachycardia with block

◆ Rhythm
 – Atrial: Regular.
 – Ventricular: Regular if block is constant, irregular if block is variable.
◆ Rate
 – Atrial: 140 to 250 beats/minute and a multiple of ventricular rate.
 – Ventricular: Varies with block.
◆ P wave
 – Slightly abnormal.

◆ PR interval
 – Usually constant for conducted P waves.
 – May vary.
◆ QRS complex
 – Usually normal.
◆ T wave
 – Usually indiscernible.
◆ QT interval
 – May be indiscernible.
◆ Other
 – More than one P wave for each QRS.

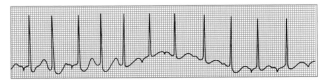

ECG characteristics of multifocal atrial tachycardia

◆ Rhythm
 – Atrial: Irregular.
 – Ventricular: Irregular.
◆ Rate
 – Atrial: 100 to 250 beats/minute (usually less than 160 beats/minute).
 – Ventricular: 100 to 250 beats/minute.
◆ P wave
 – Configuration: Varies.
 – Usually at least three different P-wave shapes must appear.

◆ PR interval
 – Varies.
◆ QRS complex
 – Usually normal.
 – May become aberrant if arrhythmia persists.
◆ T wave
 – Usually distorted.
◆ QT interval
 – May be indiscernible.
◆ Other
 – None.

(continued)

Types of atrial tachycardia *(continued)*

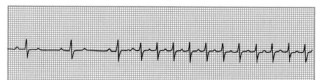

ECG characteristics of paroxysmal atrial tachycardia

◆ Rhythm
 – Atrial: Regular.
 – Ventricular: Regular.
◆ Rate
 – Atrial: 140 to 250 beats/minute.
 – Ventricular: 140 to 250 beats/minute.
◆ P wave
 – May be inverted or retrograde.
 – May not be visible.
 – May be difficult to distinguish from preceding T wave.

◆ PR interval
 – May not be measurable if P wave can't be distinguished from preceding T wave.
◆ QRS complex
 – May be aberrantly conducted.
◆ T wave
 – Usually indistinguishable.
◆ QT interval
 – May be indistinguishable.
◆ Other
 – Sudden onset, typically started by premature atrial contraction; may start and stop abruptly.

Causes

- ◆ In a normal heart:
  - Alcohol use.
  - Digoxin toxicity (most common).
  - Drug use, such as albuterol, caffeine, cocaine, marijuana, theophylline.
  - Electrolyte imbalance.
  - Hypoxia.
  - Physical stress.
  - Psychological stress.
- ◆ In primary or secondary cardiac disorders:
  - Cardiomyopathy.
  - Congenital anomalies.
  - Myocardial infarction (MI).
  - Valvular heart disease.
  - Wolff-Parkinson-White (WPW) syndrome.
- ◆ May be a component of sick sinus syndrome.
- ◆ Other causes:
  - Cor pulmonale.
  - Hyperthyroidism.
  - Systemic hypertension.

Clinical significance

◆ If nonsustained, usually benign in a healthy person.
◆ May precede more serious ventricular arrhythmias, especially if patient has heart disease.
◆ May cause the following from increased ventricular rate:
 – Decreased ventricular filling time.
 – Increased myocardial oxygen consumption.
 – Decreased oxygen supply to the myocardium.
◆ May lead to heart failure, myocardial ischemia, and MI.

Signs and symptoms

◆ Rapid apical pulse rate.
◆ Rapid peripheral pulse rate.
◆ Regular or irregular rhythm, depending on type of atrial tachycardia.
◆ Sudden feeling of palpitations, especially with PAT.
◆ Decreased cardiac output and possible hypotension and syncope from persistent tachycardia and rapid ventricular rate.

Interventions

◆ Treatment depends on the type of tachycardia and the severity of symptoms.

◆ Inquire about digoxin use, assess the patient for evidence of digoxin toxicity, and monitor digoxin blood levels.

◆ Valsalva's maneuver or carotid sinus massage may be used to treat PAT.

 RED FLAG *If vagal maneuvers are used, keep resuscitative equipment readily available because vagal stimulation can cause bradycardia, ventricular arrhythmias, and asystole.*

◆ Drug therapy (pharmacologic cardioversion) may be used to increase the degree of atrioventricular block and decrease the ventricular response rate. Appropriate drugs include the following:
  – Amiodarone.
  – Beta blockers.
  – Calcium channel blockers.
  – Digoxin.

◆ If other treatments fail or the patient is unstable, synchronized electrical cardioversion may be used.

◆ Atrial overdrive pacing may stop the arrhythmia by suppressing spontaneous depolarization of the ectopic pacemaker with a series of paced electrical impulses.

◆ If the arrhythmia is related to WPW syndrome, catheter ablation may control recurrent episodes of PAT.

◆ Because MAT typically occurs in patients with chronic pulmonary disease, the rhythm may not respond to treatment.

 RED FLAG *Assess the patient for chest pain, evidence of decreased cardiac output, and evidence of heart failure or myocardial ischemia.*

Tachycardia algorithm

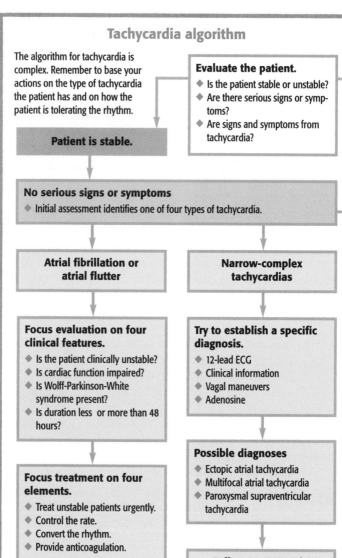

The algorithm for tachycardia is complex. Remember to base your actions on the type of tachycardia the patient has and on how the patient is tolerating the rhythm.

Evaluate the patient.
- Is the patient stable or unstable?
- Are there serious signs or symptoms?
- Are signs and symptoms from tachycardia?

Patient is stable.

No serious signs or symptoms
- Initial assessment identifies one of four types of tachycardia.

Atrial fibrillation or atrial flutter

Narrow-complex tachycardias

Focus evaluation on four clinical features.
- Is the patient clinically unstable?
- Is cardiac function impaired?
- Is Wolff-Parkinson-White syndrome present?
- Is duration less or more than 48 hours?

Try to establish a specific diagnosis.
- 12-lead ECG
- Clinical information
- Vagal maneuvers
- Adenosine

Possible diagnoses
- Ectopic atrial tachycardia
- Multifocal atrial tachycardia
- Paroxysmal supraventricular tachycardia

Focus treatment on four elements.
- Treat unstable patients urgently.
- Control the rate.
- Convert the rhythm.
- Provide anticoagulation.

Follow treatment in narrow-complex tachycardia algorithm.

Follow treatment in atrial fibrillation section and in atrial flutter text.

Patient is unstable.

Serious signs or symptoms
◆ Signs and symptoms result from rapid heart rate (greater than 150 beats/minute). Prepare for immediate cardioversion.

Stable wide-complex tachycardia of unknown type

Stable monomorphic or polymorphic ventricular tachycardia. (See stable monomorphic or polymorphic ventricular tachycardia algorithm.)

Try to establish a specific diagnosis.
◆ 12-lead ECG
◆ Esophageal lead
◆ Clinical information

Confirmed stable ventricular tachycardia
(See stable monomorphic or polymorphic ventricular tachycardia algorithm.)

Confirmed supraventricular tachycardia

Wide-complex tachycardia of unknown type

Preserved cardiac function

Impaired heart (ejection fraction < 40%), clinical heart failure

Cardioversion, procainamide, or amiodarone

Cardioversion or amiodarone

Narrow-complex tachycardia algorithm

Types of narrow-complex tachycardia include junctional tachycardia, paroxysmal supraventricular tachycardia (PSVT), and multifocal atrial tachycardia (MAT). Treatment for each type of rhythm depends on how well the patient tolerates the rhythm.

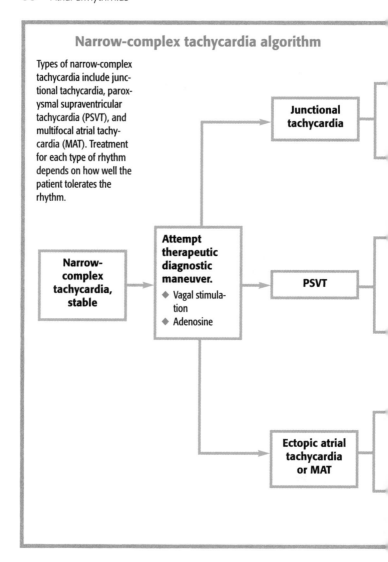

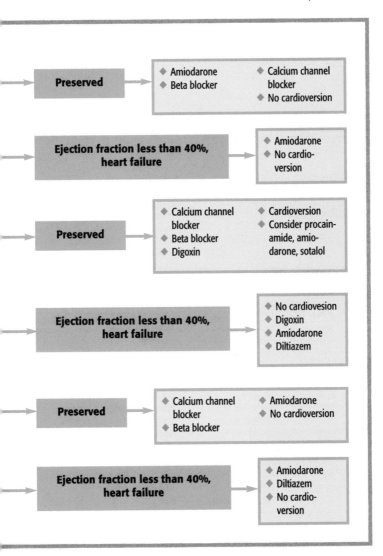

Preserved
- Amiodarone
- Beta blocker
- Calcium channel blocker
- No cardioversion

Ejection fraction less than 40%, heart failure
- Amiodarone
- No cardio-version

Preserved
- Calcium channel blocker
- Beta blocker
- Digoxin
- Cardioversion
- Consider procain-amide, amio-darone, sotalol

Ejection fraction less than 40%, heart failure
- No cardiovesion
- Digoxin
- Amiodarone
- Diltiazem

Preserved
- Calcium channel blocker
- Beta blocker
- Amiodarone
- No cardioversion

Ejection fraction less than 40%, heart failure
- Amiodarone
- Diltiazem
- No cardio-version

Atrial flutter

♦ A supraventricular tachycardia.
♦ Atrial rate: 250 to 400 beats/minute (usually about 300 beats/minute).

Recognizing atrial flutter

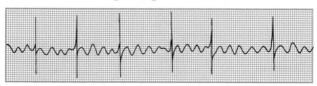

ECG characteristics

♦ Rhythm
 – Atrial: Regular.
 – Ventricular: Commonly regular, although cycles may alternate (depends on atrioventricular [AV] conduction pattern).
♦ Rate
 – Atrial: 250 to 400 beats/minute.
 – Ventricular: Usually 60 to 100 beats/minute (one-half to one-fourth of atrial rate), but may be 125 to 150 beats/minute depending on degree of AV block.
 – Usually expressed as ratio (2:1 or 4:1, for example).
 – Commonly 150 beats/minute ventricular and 300 beats/minute atrial, known as 2:1 block.
 – Every second, third, or fourth impulse conducted to ventricles because AV node usually won't accept more than 180 impulses/minute.
 – When atrial flutter first recognized, ventricular rate usually exceeds 100 beats/minute.

♦ P wave
 – Abnormal.
 – Sawtooth appearance known as flutter or F waves.
♦ PR interval
 – Not measurable.
♦ QRS complex
 – Duration: Usually within normal limits.
 – May be widened if flutter waves are buried within the complex.
♦ T wave
 – Not identifiable.
♦ QT interval
 – Not measurable because T wave isn't identifiable.
♦ Other
 – Atrial rhythm may vary between a fibrillatory line and flutter waves (called atrial fib-flutter), with an irregular ventricular response.
 – May be difficult to differentiate atrial flutter from atrial fibrillation.

- Originates in a single atrial focus.
- Results from a reentrant circuit and possibly increased automaticity.

Causes

- Conditions that enlarge atrial tissue and elevate atrial pressures.
- Other causes:
    - Cardiac surgery with acute myocardial infarction.
    - Chronic obstructive pulmonary disease.
    - Digoxin toxicity.
    - Hyperthyroidism.
    - Mitral valve disease.
    - Pericardial disease.
    - Primary myocardial disease.
    - Systemic arterial hypoxia.
    - Tricuspid valve disease.

Clinical significance

◆ Determined by number of impulses conducted through atrioventricular (AV) node (expressed as a conduction ratio with
  ventricular rate forming second number, such as 2:1 or 4:1).
◆ Serious compromise to cardiac output if ventricular rate is
  too slow (less than 40 beats/minute) or too fast (more than
  150 beats/minute).
◆ Increasing danger with increasing ventricular rate.
◆ Reduced ventricular filling time and coronary perfusion from
  rapid ventricular rate, possibly resulting in these conditions:
    – Angina.
    – Heart failure.
    – Hypotension.
    – Pulmonary edema.
    – Syncope.

Signs and symptoms

◆ Possibly none if ventricular rate is normal.
◆ Feeling of palpitations if ventricular rate is rapid.
◆ Evidence of reduced cardiac output if ventricular rate is rapid.

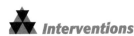 *Interventions*

◆ Interventions depend on the patient's cardiac function, preexcitation syndromes, and duration of the arrhythmia (less or more than 48 hours).

◆ If the patient is hemodynamically unstable and atrial flutter has lasted 48 hours or less, synchronized electrical cardioversion or countershock should be performed right away.

◆ If atrial flutter has lasted more than 48 hours, electrical cardioversion won't be performed unless the patient is adequately anticoagulated because of the increased risk of thromboembolism.

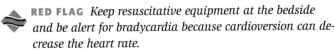 RED FLAG *Keep resuscitative equipment at the bedside and be alert for bradycardia because cardioversion can decrease the heart rate.*

◆ Ventricular rate can be controlled with drugs that block the AV node, such as calcium channel blockers and beta blockers.

◆ Be alert to the effects of digoxin, which depresses the SA node.

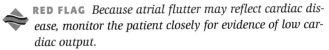 RED FLAG *Because atrial flutter may reflect cardiac disease, monitor the patient closely for evidence of low cardiac output.*

◆ Recurrent atrial flutter may be treated with ablation therapy.

Atrial fibrillation

◆ Chaotic, asynchronous, electrical activity in atrial tissue.
◆ Results from firing of multiple impulses from numerous ectopic pacemakers in the atria.
◆ Absence of P waves.
◆ Irregularly irregular ventricular response.
◆ May be preceded by premature atrial contractions.

Recognizing atrial fibrillation

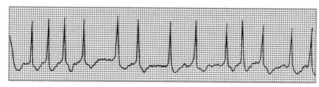

ECG characteristics

◆ Rhythm
 – Atrial: Irregularly irregular.
 – Ventricular: Irregularly irregular.
◆ Rate
 – Atrial: Almost indiscernible, usually above 400 beats/minute, and far exceeding ventricular rate because most impulses aren't conducted through the AV junction.
 – Ventricular: Usually 100 to 150 beats/minute but can be below 100 beats/minute.
◆ P wave
 – Absent
 – Replaced by baseline fibrillatory (f) waves that represent atrial tetanization from rapid atrial depolarizations.

◆ PR interval
 – Indiscernible.
◆ QRS complex
 – Duration and configuration usually normal.
◆ T wave
 – Indiscernible.
◆ QT interval
 – Not measurable.
◆ Other
 – Atrial rhythm may vary between fibrillatory line and flutter waves, called atrial fib-flutter.
 – May be difficult to differentiate atrial fibrillation from multifocal atrial tachycardia and junctional rhythm.

Causes

◆ Acute myocardial infarction.
◆ Atrial septal defect.
◆ Cardiac surgery.
◆ Cardiomyopathy.
◆ Chronic obstructive pulmonary disease.
◆ Coronary artery disease.
◆ Drugs, such as aminophylline and digoxin.
◆ Endogenous catecholamine released during exercise.
◆ Hypertension.
◆ Hyperthyroidism.
◆ In a healthy person, smoking, drinking coffee or alcohol, or fatigue or stress.
◆ Pericarditis.
◆ Rheumatic heart disease.
◆ Valvular heart disease (especially mitral valve disease).

Clinical significance

◆ Decrease in normal end-diastolic volume (by about 20%) from loss of atrial kick.
◆ Decreased diastolic filling time from rapid heart rate.
◆ Significant reduction in cardiac output.
◆ Heart failure, myocardial ischemia, or syncope if atrial fibrillation uncontrolled.
◆ Possible severe heart failure if patient has cardiac disease, such as hypertrophic cardiomyopathy, mitral stenosis, rheumatic heart disease, or prosthetic mitral valve.

 RED FLAG *Untreated atrial fibrillation can lead to cardiovascular collapse, thrombus formation, pulmonary embolism, and thromboembolic stroke.*

◆ May be difficult to distinguish from multifocal atrial tachycardia.

Signs and symptoms

♦ Irregularly irregular pulse rhythm with normal or abnormal heart rate.
♦ Radial pulse rate slower than apical pulse rate.
♦ Palpable peripheral pulse only with stronger contractions, not with weaker ones of atrial fibrillation.
♦ Evidence of decreased cardiac output, such as hypotension and light-headedness, with new-onset atrial fibrillation and a rapid ventricular rate.
♦ Possibly no symptoms in chronic atrial fibrillation, in which patient may be able to compensate for decreased cardiac output, but an increased risk of pulmonary, cerebral, or other thromboembolic events.

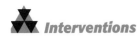 *Interventions*

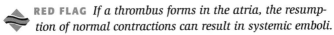

◆ Interventions aim to reduce the ventricular response rate to less than 100 beats/minute, establish anticoagulation, and restore and maintain a sinus rhythm.

◆ Treatment typically includes drug therapy to control the ventricular response or a combination of electrical cardioversion and drug therapy.

◆ If the patient is hemodynamically unstable, synchronized electrical cardioversion should be performed right away. It's most successful if done within 48 hours after atrial fibrillation starts.

◆ A transesophageal echocardiogram may be obtained before cardioversion to rule out thrombi in the atria.

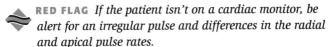 **RED FLAG** *If a thrombus forms in the atria, the resumption of normal contractions can result in systemic emboli.*

◆ Beta blockers and calcium channel blockers are the drugs of choice to control the ventricular rate. Patients with reduced left ventricular function typically receive digoxin.

◆ Anticoagulation is crucial in reducing the risk of thromboembolism. Warfarin and heparin are used for anticoagulation and to prepare the patient for elective cardioversion.

◆ Symptomatic atrial fibrillation that doesn't respond to routine treatment may be treated with radiofrequency ablation therapy.

◆ Monitor peripheral and apical pulses; watch for evidence of decreased cardiac output and heart failure.

RED FLAG *If the patient isn't on a cardiac monitor, be alert for an irregular pulse and differences in the radial and apical pulse rates.*

◆ If drug therapy is used, monitor serum drug levels and watch for evidence of toxicity.

◆ Tell the patient to report changes in pulse rate, dizziness, feeling faint, chest pain, and signs of heart failure, such as dyspnea and peripheral edema.

Distinguishing atrial fibrillation from atrial flutter

It isn't uncommon for atrial flutter to have an irregular pattern of impulse conduction to the ventricles. In some leads, this may be confused with atrial fibrillation. Here's how to tell the two arrhythmias apart.

Atrial fibrillation

◆ Fibrillatory waves (f waves) occur in an irregular pattern, making the atrial rhythm irregular.
◆ If you see atrial activity on the rhythm strip that in some places looks like flutter waves and seems to be regular for a short time, and in other places looks like fibrillatory waves, interpret the rhythm as atrial fibrillation. Coarse fibrillatory waves may sometimes have the characteristic sawtooth appearance of flutter waves.

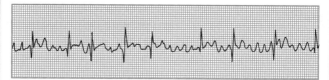

Atrial flutter

◆ Look for characteristic abnormal P waves that produce a sawtooth appearance, known as flutter waves, or F waves. These can be identified most easily in leads I, II, and V_1.
◆ Remember that the atrial rhythm is regular. You should be able to map the F waves across the rhythm strip. Although some F waves may occur within the QRS or T waves, subsequent F waves will be visible and will occur on time.

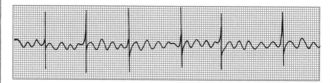

Distinguishing atrial fibrillation from multifocal atrial tachycardia

To help you decide whether a rhythm is atrial fibrillation or the similar multifocal atrial tachycardia (MAT), focus on the P waves and the atrial and ventricular rhythms. You may find it helpful to look at a rhythm strip that's longer than 6 seconds.

Atrial fibrillation

◆ Carefully look for discernible P waves before each QRS complex.

◆ If you can't clearly identify P waves, and if fibrillatory (f) waves appear in place of P waves, then the rhythm is probably atrial fibrillation.

◆ Carefully look at the rhythm, focusing on the R-R intervals. One of the hallmarks of atrial fibrillation is an irregularly irregular rhythm.

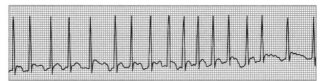

Multifocal atrial tachycardia

◆ P waves are present in MAT. Keep in mind, though, that at least three different P-wave shapes will be visible in a single rhythm strip.

◆ You should be able to see most or all of the P-wave shapes repeat.

◆ Although the atrial and ventricular rhythms are irregular, the irregularity usually isn't as pronounced as in atrial fibrillation.

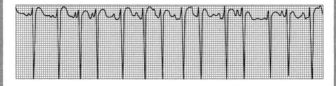

Ashman's phenomenon

♦ Aberrant conduction of premature supraventricular beats to the ventricles.
♦ A benign phenomenon.
♦ Commonly occurs with atrial fibrillation, but may occur with any arrhythmia that affects R-R interval.
♦ Abnormal beat usually occurs as right bundle-branch block because normal refractory period for the right bundle branch is slightly longer than the left, so premature beats more commonly reach the right bundle when it's partly or fully refractory.

Ashman's phenomenon

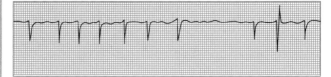

ECG characteristics

♦ Rhythm
  – Atrial: Irregular.
  – Ventricular: Irregular.
♦ Rate
  – Reflects the underlying rhythm.
♦ P wave
  – May be visible.
  – Abnormal configuration.
  – Unchanged if present in the underlying rhythm.
♦ PR interval
  – Commonly changes on the premature beat, if measurable at all.
♦ QRS complex
  – Altered configuration with right bundle-branch block pattern.

♦ T wave
  – Deflection opposite that of QRS complex in most leads because of right bundle-branch block.
♦ QT interval
  – Usually changed because of right bundle-branch block.
♦ Other
  – No compensatory pause after an aberrant beat.
  – Aberrancy may continue for several beats and typically ends a short cycle preceded by a long cycle.

Causes

◆ A prolonged refractory period in a slower rhythm.
◆ A short cycle followed by a long cycle because the refractory period varies with the length of the cycle.

Clinical significance

◆ The importance of recognizing aberrantly conducted beats is mainly to prevent misdiagnosis and mistaken treatment of ventricular ectopy.

Signs and symptoms

◆ No signs or symptoms.

 ## Interventions

◆ No interventions are needed for this arrhythmia, although they may be needed for accompanying arrhythmias.

Wandering pacemaker

◆ Also called wandering atrial pacemaker.
◆ A shifting site of impulse formation from the sinoatrial (SA) node to another area above the ventricles — the atria or atrioventricular (AV) junctional tissue.
◆ Variable P wave and PR interval from beat to beat as pacemaker site changes.

Recognizing wandering pacemaker

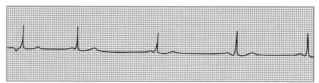

ECG characteristics

◆ Rhythm
    – Atrial: Varies slightly, with an irregular P-P interval.
    – Ventricular: Varies slightly, with an irregular R-R interval.
◆ Rate
    – Varies, but usually within normal limits or less than 60 beats/ minute.
◆ P wave
    – Altered size and configuration from changing pacemaker site.
    – May be absent, inverted, or after QRS complex if impulse originates in atrioventricular (AV) junction.
    – Appear in variable combinations with at least three different P-wave shapes visible.

◆ PR interval
    – Varies from beat to beat as pacemaker site changes.
    – May be normal or shortened when P wave present.
    – Usually less than 0.20 second.
    – Less than 0.12 second if impulse originates in AV junction.
    – Slightly irregular R-R interval from variation in PR interval.
◆ QRS complex
    – Duration and configuration usually normal because ventricular depolarization is normal.
◆ T wave
    – Normal size and configuration.
◆ QT interval
    – Usually within normal limits, but may vary.
◆ Other
    – May be difficult to differentiate wandering pacemaker from premature atrial contractions.

Causes

◆ Increased parasympathetic (vagal) influences on the SA node or AV junction.
◆ Other causes:
   – Chronic obstructive pulmonary disease.
   – Digoxin toxicity.
   – Inflammation of atrial tissue.
   – Valvular heart disease.

Clinical significance

◆ May be normal in young patients.
◆ Common in athletes with slow heart rates.
◆ Typically transient.
◆ May be difficult to distinguish from premature atrial contractions.

Signs and symptoms

◆ Usually no symptoms.
◆ Commonly no awareness of arrhythmia on patient's part.
◆ Pulse rate normal or less than 60 beats/minute.
◆ Rhythm regular or slightly irregular.

 ## Interventions

◆ Usually, no treatment is needed if the patient has no symptoms.
◆ If the patient has symptoms, medications should be reviewed and the underlying cause of the arrhythmia investigated and treated.
◆ Monitor the patient's heart rhythm.
◆ Observe the patient for evidence of hemodynamic instability, such as hypotension and changes in mental status.

Distinguishing wandering pacemaker from premature atrial contractions

Because premature atrial contractions (PACs) are common, you may miss a wandering pacemaker rhythm unless you examine the rhythm strip carefully. You may find it helpful to look at a rhythm strip that's longer than 6 seconds.

Wandering pacemaker

◆ Carefully examine the P waves. You'll be able to identify at least three different shapes of P waves (see shaded areas below) in wandering pacemaker.

◆ The atrial rhythm varies slightly, with an irregular P-P interval. The ventricular rhythm varies slightly as well, with an irregular R-R interval. These slight variations result from the changing site of impulse formation.

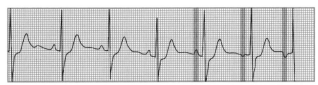

Premature atrial contractions

◆ The PAC occurs earlier than the sinus P wave, with an abnormal configuration when compared with a sinus P wave (see shaded area below).

◆ It's possible, although rare, to see multifocal PACs that originate from multiple ectopic pacemaker sites in the atria. If this happens, the P waves may have different shapes.

◆ Except for the irregular atrial and ventricular rhythms that result from the PAC, the underlying rhythm is usually regular.

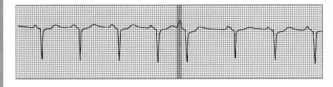

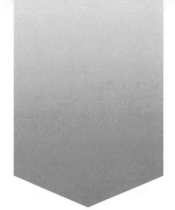

4

Junctional arrhythmias

Premature junctional contractions

◆ Junctional (ectopic) beats that occur before normal sinus beats and interrupt the underlying rhythm.

◆ Impulses generated in the atrioventricular (AV) junction.

◆ Commonly result from enhanced automaticity in junctional tissue or bundle of His.

◆ Atria depolarized in a retrograde fashion, causing an inverted P wave.

◆ Ventricles depolarized normally.

Recognizing premature junctional contractions

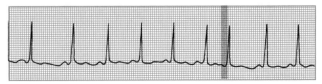

ECG characteristics

◆ Rhythm
- Atrial: Irregular during premature junctional contractions (PJCs).
- Ventricular: Irregular during PJCs.
- Underlying rhythm may be regular.

◆ Rate
- Atrial: Reflects underlying rhythm.
- Ventricular: Reflects underlying rhythm.

◆ P wave
- Usually inverted (leads II, III, and aV$_F$).
- May occur before, during, or after QRS complex, depending on initial direction of depolarization.
- May be absent.
- May be hidden in the QRS complex.

◆ PR interval
- Shortened (less than 0.12 second) if P wave precedes QRS complex.
- Not measurable if no P wave precedes QRS complex.

◆ QRS complex
- Usually normal configuration and duration (less than 0.12 second) because ventricles usually depolarize normally.

◆ T wave
- Usually normal configuration.

◆ QT interval
- Usually within normal limits.

◆ Other
- Commonly accompanied by a compensatory pause reflecting retrograde atrial conduction.

Locating the P wave

When specialized pacemaker cells in the atrioventricular junction take over as the dominant pacemaker of the heart, several events can occur:
◆ Atrial depolarization can precede ventricular depolarization.
◆ Ventricular depolarization can precede atrial depolarization.
◆ Atrial and ventricular depolarization can occur simultaneously.
   These illustrations show the various locations of P waves in junctional arrhythmias, depending on the direction of depolarization.

If the atria are depolarized first, the P wave will appear before the QRS complex.

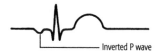

Inverted P wave

If the ventricles are depolarized first, the P wave will appear after the QRS complex.

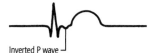

Inverted P wave

If the ventricles and atria are depolarized simultaneously, the P wave will be hidden in the QRS complex.

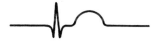

Causes

◆ Chronic obstructive pulmonary disease.
◆ Coronary artery disease.
◆ Digoxin toxicity.
◆ Electrolyte imbalances.
◆ Excessive alcohol intake.
◆ Excessive caffeine intake.
◆ Excessive nicotine intake.
◆ Heart failure.
◆ Hyperthyroidism.
◆ Inflammatory changes in the AV junction after heart surgery.
◆ Myocardial ischemia.
◆ Pericarditis.
◆ Stress.
◆ Valvular heart disease.

Clinical significance

◆ Usually harmless unless frequent (more than six per minute).

 RED FLAG *Frequent premature junctional contractions (PJCs) indicate junctional irritability and can lead to a more serious arrhythmia, such as junctional tachycardia. In patients taking digoxin, PJCs are a common early sign of toxicity.*

Signs and symptoms

◆ Usually no symptoms.
◆ Possible feeling of palpitations or skipped beats.
◆ Hypotension from a transient decrease in cardiac output if PJCs are frequent enough.

 Interventions

◆ PJCs usually need no treatment if the patient has no symptoms.
◆ If the patient has symptoms, the underlying cause should be treated.
◆ If the patient has digoxin toxicity, stop the drug and monitor the patient's drug levels.
◆ Monitor the patient for hemodynamic instability.
◆ If ectopic beats occur frequently because of caffeine, the patient should decrease or eliminate caffeine intake.

Junctional rhythm

◆ Also known as junctional escape rhythm.
◆ Originates in the atrioventricular (AV) junction when a higher pacemaker site in the atria, usually the sinoatrial (SA) node, fails as the dominant pacemaker, possibly for one of these reasons:
  – Firing rate of higher pacemaker sites falls below intrinsic firing rate of AV junction.
  – Pacemaker fails to generate an impulse.
  – Impulse conduction is blocked.

Recognizing a junctional rhythm

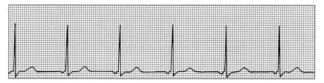

ECG characteristics

◆ Rhythm
  – Atrial: Regular.
  – Ventricular: Regular.
◆ Rate
  – Atrial: 40 to 60 beats/minute.
  – Ventricular: 40 to 60 beats/minute.
◆ P wave
  – Usually inverted (leads II, III, and aV$_F$).
  – May occur before or after QRS complex
  – May be hidden in QRS complex.
  – May be absent.

◆ PR interval
  – Shortened (less than 0.12 second) if P wave precedes QRS complex.
  – Not measurable if no P wave precedes QRS complex.
◆ QRS complex
  – Duration usually within normal limits.
  – Configuration usually normal.
◆ T wave
  – Configuration usually normal.
◆ QT interval
  – Usually within normal limits.
◆ Other
  – May be difficult to differentiate between junctional rhythm and idioventricular rhythm.

◆ Atria are depolarized by retrograde conduction.
◆ Normal conduction through ventricles.
◆ Intrinsic firing rate for cells in AV junction: 40 to 60 beats/minute.

Causes

◆ A condition that disturbs normal SA node function or impulse conduction.
◆ Specific causes:
  – Cardiomyopathy.
  – Electrolyte imbalance.
  – Heart failure.
  – Hypoxia.
  – Increased parasympathetic (vagal) tone.
  – Myocarditis.
  – SA node ischemia.
  – Sick sinus syndrome.
  – Valvular heart disease.
◆ Drug-related causes:
  – Beta blockers.
  – Calcium channel blockers.
  – Digoxin.

Clinical significance

◆ Protects the heart from potentially life-threatening idioventricular rhythms.
◆ Significance based on the patient's ability to tolerate decreased heart rate (40 to 60 beats/minute), decreased cardiac output, and underlying cardiac disease.
◆ May be difficult to distinguish from accelerated idioventricular rhythm.

Signs and symptoms

◆ May be no symptoms.
◆ Slow, regular pulse rate of 40 to 60 beats/minute.

 RED FLAG *Pulse rates below 60 beats/minute may lead to inadequate cardiac output, causing hypotension, syncope, or blurred vision.*

 Interventions

 RED FLAG *Because a junctional rhythm can prevent ventricular standstill, it should never be suppressed.*

◆ Treatment for a junctional rhythm involves identification and correction of the underlying cause, whenever possible.
◆ Atropine may be used to increase the heart rate, or a transcutaneous, temporary, or permanent pacemaker may be used.
◆ Monitor the patient's digoxin and electrolyte levels.
◆ Watch for evidence of decreased cardiac output, such as hypotension, syncope, and blurred vision.

Distinguishing a junctional rhythm from an accelerated idioventricular rhythm

A junctional rhythm and an accelerated Idioventricular rhythm appear similar but have different causes. To distinguish between them, closely examine the duration of the QRS complex, and then look for P waves.

Junctional rhythm

◆ The QRS complex duration and configuration are usually normal.

◆ Inverted P waves typically appear before or after the QRS complex, although P waves may be absent or buried in the QRS complex.

◆ The ventricular rate usually is 40 to 60 beats/minute.

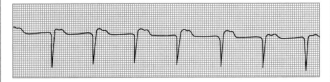

Accelerated idioventricular rhythm

◆ The QRS complex duration will be greater than 0.12 second.

◆ The QRS complex will have a wide and bizarre configuration.

◆ P waves usually are absent.

◆ The ventricular rate usually is 40 to 100 beats/minute.

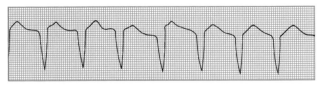

Accelerated junctional rhythm

◆ Originates in the atrioventricular (AV) junction.
◆ Involves enhanced automaticity of AV junctional tissue.
◆ Occurs at 60 to 100 beats/minute (accelerated), exceeding the inherent junctional rate of 40 to 60 beats/minute.
◆ Not considered junctional tachycardia because rate is below 100 beats/minute.
◆ Atria depolarized by retrograde conduction.
◆ Ventricles depolarized normally.

Recognizing an accelerated junctional rhythm

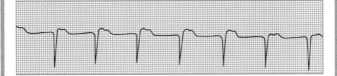

ECG characteristics

◆ Rhythm
  – Atrial: Regular.
  – Ventricular: Regular.
◆ Rate
  – Atrial: 60 to 100 beats/minute.
  – Ventricular: 60 to 100 beats/minute.
◆ P wave
  – If present, inverted in leads II, III, and aV$_F$.
  – May occur before, during, or after QRS complex.
  – May be hidden in QRS complex.
  – May be absent.

◆ PR interval
  – Shortened (less than 0.12 second) if P wave precedes QRS complex.
  – Not measurable if no P wave precedes QRS complex.
◆ QRS complex
  – Duration: Usually within normal limits, but may be slightly prolonged.
  – Configuration: Usually normal.
◆ T wave
  – Usually within normal limits.
◆ QT interval
  – Usually within normal limits.
◆ Other
  – None.

Causes

♦ Cardiac surgery.
♦ Digoxin toxicity (common cause).
♦ Electrolyte disturbance.
♦ Heart failure.
♦ Inferior-wall myocardial infarction (MI).
♦ Myocarditis.
♦ Posterior-wall MI.
♦ Rheumatic heart disease.
♦ Valvular heart disease.

Clinical significance

♦ Decreased cardiac output (from loss of atrial kick) if atrial depolarization occurs after or simultaneously with ventricular depolarization.

Signs and symptoms

♦ Normal pulse rate and regular rhythm.
♦ May be no symptoms because accelerated junctional rhythm has the same rate as sinus rhythm.
♦ May be symptoms of decreased cardiac output, such as hypotension, changes in mental status, and weak peripheral pulses.

 Interventions

♦ Treatment for accelerated junctional rhythm involves identifying and correcting the underlying cause.
♦ Assess the patient for signs and symptoms of decreased cardiac output and hemodynamic instability.
♦ Monitor serum digoxin and electrolyte levels.

Junctional tachycardia

- ◆ Three or more premature junctional contractions in a row.
- ◆ A supraventricular tachycardia.
- ◆ Usually from enhanced automaticity of the atrioventricular (AV) junction, which causes the AV junction to override the sinoatrial node as the dominant pacemaker.
- ◆ Atria depolarized by retrograde conduction.
- ◆ Normal conduction through the ventricles.
- ◆ Rate: Usually 100 to 200 beats/minute.

Recognizing junctional tachycardia

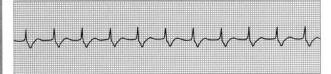

ECG characteristics

- ◆ Rhythm
  - – Atrial: Usually regular, but may be difficult to determine if P wave is absent or hidden in QRS complex or preceding T wave.
  - – Ventricular: Usually regular.
- ◆ Rate
  - – Atrial: Exceeds 100 beats/minute (usually 100 to 200 beats/minute), but may be difficult to determine if P wave is absent or hidden in QRS complex.
  - – Ventricular: Exceeds 100 beats/minute (usually 100 to 200 beats/minute).
- ◆ P wave
  - – Usually inverted in leads II, III, and aV$_F$.
  - – May occur before or after QRS complex.
  - – May be hidden in QRS complex.
  - – May be absent.

- ◆ PR interval
  - – Shortened (less than 0.12 second) if P wave precedes QRS complex.
  - – Not measurable if no P wave precedes QRS complex.
- ◆ QRS complex
  - – Duration: Within normal limits.
  - – Configuration: Usually normal.
- ◆ T wave
  - – Configuration: Usually normal.
  - – May be abnormal if P wave is hidden in T wave.
  - – May be indiscernible because of fast rate.
- ◆ QT interval
  - – Usually within normal limits.
- ◆ Other
  - – None.

Causes

◆ Digoxin toxicity (most common).
◆ Electrolyte imbalance.
◆ Heart failure.
◆ Hypokalemia (may aggravate condition).
◆ Inferior-wall myocardial infarction.
◆ Inferior-wall myocardial ischemia.
◆ Inflammation of AV junction following heart surgery.
◆ Posterior-wall myocardial infarction.
◆ Posterior-wall myocardial ischemia.
◆ Valvular heart disease.

Clinical significance

◆ Depends on rate, underlying cause, and patient's tolerance for tachycardia.
◆ Higher ventricular rates: Decreased cardiac output from decreasing ventricular filling time.
◆ Loss of atrial kick if atrial depolarization occurs after or simultaneously with ventricular depolarization.

Signs and symptoms

◆ Pulse rate above 100 beats/minute with a regular rhythm.

 RED FLAG *A patient with a rapid heart rate may experience the effects of decreased cardiac output and hemodynamic instability, including hypotension.*

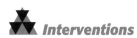 *Interventions*

◆ The underlying cause should be identified and treated.

◆ If the cause is digoxin toxicity, the drug should be discontinued.

◆ In some cases of digoxin toxicity, a digoxin-binding drug may be used to reduce serum digoxin levels.

◆ Vagal maneuvers and drugs such as adenosine may slow the heart rate for a symptomatic patient.

◆ A patient with recurrent junctional tachycardia may be treated with ablation therapy followed by permanent pacemaker insertion.

◆ Watch for evidence of decreased cardiac output.

◆ Check digoxin and potassium levels, and give potassium supplements as needed.

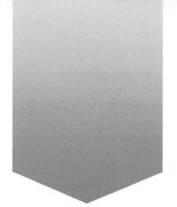

5

Ventricular arrhythmias

Premature ventricular contractions

◆ Ectopic beats that originate in the ventricles and occur earlier than expected.
◆ May occur singly, in pairs (couplets), and in clusters.
◆ May appear in patterns, such as bigeminy or trigeminy.
◆ Commonly followed by a compensatory pause.
◆ May be uniform in appearance, arising from a single ectopic ventricular pacemaker site.
◆ May be multiform, originating from a single pacemaker site but with QRS complexes that differ in size, shape, and direction.
◆ May be unifocal or multifocal.
  – Unifocal: Originate from the same ventricular ectopic pacemaker site.
  – Multifocal: Originate from different ectopic pacemaker sites in the ventricles.

Recognizing premature ventricular contractions

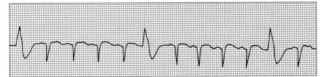

ECG characteristics

◆ Rhythm
- Atrial: Irregular during premature ventricular contractions (PVCs).
- Ventricular: Irregular during PVCs.
- Underlying rhythm may be regular.

◆ Rate
- Atrial: Reflects underlying rhythm.
- Ventricular: Reflects underlying rhythm.

◆ P wave
- Usually absent in ectopic beat.
- May appear after QRS complex with retrograde conduction to atria.
- Usually normal if present in underlying rhythm.

◆ PR interval
- Not measurable except in underlying rhythm.

◆ QRS complex
- Earlier than expected.
- Duration: Exceeds 0.12 second.
- Configuration: Bizarre and wide, but usually normal in underlying rhythm.

◆ T wave
- Opposite direction to QRS complex.
- May trigger more serious rhythm disturbances when PVC occurs on the down slope of preceding normal T wave (R-on-T phenomenon).

◆ QT interval
- Not usually measured except in underlying rhythm.

◆ Other
- PVC may be followed by full or incomplete compensatory pause.
- Full compensatory pause plus preceding R-R interval equals sum of two R-R intervals in underlying rhythm.
- Incomplete compensatory pause: Sinoatrial (SA) node is depolarized by PVC, which resets timing of SA node.
- Incomplete compensatory pause plus preceding R-R interval is less than the sum of two R-R intervals in underlying rhythm.
- Interpolated PVC: Occurs between two normally conducted QRS complexes without great disturbance to underlying rhythm.
- Full compensatory pause absent with interpolated PVCs.
- May be difficult to distinguish PVCs from aberrant ventricular conduction.

Causes

- ◆ Enhanced automaticity in the ventricular conduction system or muscle tissue (usual cause).
- ◆ Irritable focus from disruption of normal electrolyte shifts during cellular depolarization and repolarization.
- ◆ Alcohol ingestion.
- ◆ Caffeine ingestion.
- ◆ Tobacco use.
- ◆ Drug intoxication, particularly with amphetamines, cocaine, digoxin, phenothiazines, tricyclic antidepressants.
- ◆ Electrolyte imbalance (hyperkalemia, hypocalcemia, hypomagnesemia, hypokalemia).
- ◆ Enlargement of ventricular chambers.
- ◆ Hypoxia.
- ◆ Increased sympathetic stimulation.
- ◆ Irritation of ventricles by pacemaker electrodes or a pulmonary artery catheter.
- ◆ Metabolic acidosis.
- ◆ Mitral valve prolapse.
- ◆ Myocardial infarction.
- ◆ Myocardial ischemia.
- ◆ Myocarditis.
- ◆ Sympathomimetic drugs, such as epinephrine and isoproterenol.

Clinical significance

◆ Can lead to more serious arrhythmias, such as VT or VF, especially in patients with ischemic or damaged hearts.
◆ Decreased cardiac output from:
  – Reduced ventricular diastolic filling time.
  – Loss of atrial kick for affected beat.
◆ Significance varies with duration of abnormal rhythm and body's ability to maintain adequate perfusion.
◆ May follow an abnormal conduction pathway, giving abnormal appearance to QRS complex and known as aberrancy or aberrant ventricular conduction.
◆ May be difficult to distinguish PVCs from aberrant ventricular conduction.

Signs and symptoms

◆ Usually a normal pulse rate with a momentarily irregular pulse rhythm when a premature ventricular contraction (PVC) occurs.
◆ May be no symptoms.
◆ Abnormally early heart sound with each PVC on auscultation.
◆ Feeling of palpitations if PVCs are frequent.
◆ Possible evidence of decreased cardiac output, including hypotension and syncope.

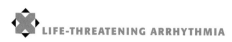

Patterns of potentially dangerous PVCs

Some premature ventricular contractions (PVCs) are more dangerous than others. Here are some potentially dangerous ones.

Paired PVCs

Two PVCs in a row, called paired PVCs or a ventricular couplet (see shaded areas), can produce ventricular tachycardia (VT). That's because the second contraction usually meets refractory tissue. A burst, or salvo, of three or more PVCs in a row is considered a run of VT.

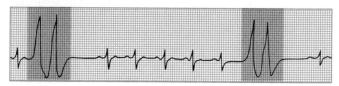

Multiform PVCs

Multiform PVCs look different from one another (see shaded areas) and arise either from different sites or from the same site via abnormal conduction. Multiform PVCs may indicate severe heart disease or digoxin toxicity.

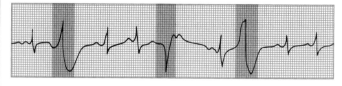

Bigeminy and trigeminy

PVCs that occur every other beat (bigeminy) or every third beat (trigeminy) can result in VT or ventricular fibrillation (VF). The shaded areas on the rhythm strip shown below illustrate ventricular bigeminy.

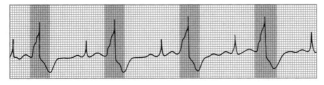

R-on-T phenomenon

In R-on-T phenomenon, a PVC occurs so early that it falls on the T wave of the preceding beat (see shaded area). Because the cells haven't fully repolarized, VT or VF can result.

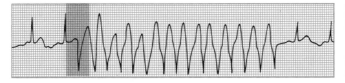

Distinguishing PVCs from ventricular aberrancy

Premature ventricular contractions (PVCs) and ventricular aberrancy present one of the most challenging lookalikes. Indeed, sometimes they can be distinguished with complete confidence only in an electrophysiology lab.

Ventricular aberrancy, or aberrant ventricular conduction, occurs when an impulse originating in the sinoatrial node, atria, or atrioventricular junction is temporarily conducted abnormally through the bundle branches. The abnormal conduction results in a bundle-branch block, usually because electrical impulses arrive at the bundle branches before the branches have been sufficiently repolarized.

To distinguish between PVCs and ventricular aberrancy, examine the deflection of the QRS complex in lead V_1. Determine whether the QRS complex is primarily positive or negative. Based on this information, follow these clues to guide your analysis.

Mostly positive QRS complex

- ◆ Right bundle-branch aberrancy will have a triphasic rSR′ configuration in V_1 and a triphasic qRS configuration in V_6.
- ◆ If there are two positive peaks in V_1 and the left peak is taller, the beat is probably a PVC.
- ◆ PVCs will be monophasic or biphasic in V_1, and biphasic in V_6, with a deep S wave.

Comparing PVC with right bundle-branch aberrancy

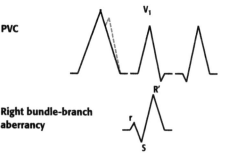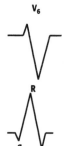

Mostly negative QRS complex

◆ Left bundle-branch aberrancy will have a narrow R wave with a quick downstroke in leads V_1 and V_2, and no Q wave in V_6.

◆ PVCs will have a wide R wave (greater than 0.03 second) and a notched or slurred S-wave downstroke in leads V_1 and V_2, with a duration greater than 0.06 second from the onset of the R wave to the deepest point of the S wave in V_1 and V_2, and a Q wave in V_6.

◆ P waves commonly precede aberrancies, and they usually don't precede PVCs.

◆ Aberrancies usually have a QRS duration of 0.12 second. PVCs are more likely to have a QRS duration of 0.14 second or more.

Comparing PVC with left bundle-branch aberrancy

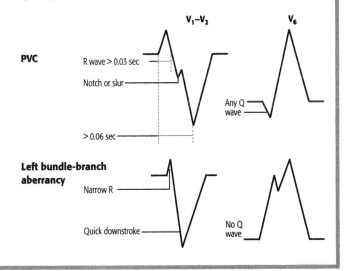

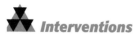 **Interventions**

◆ If the patient is asymptomatic and doesn't have heart disease, the arrhythmia probably won't need treatment.

◆ If symptoms or a dangerous form of PVC occurs, the type of treatment given will depend on the cause of the problem.

> **RED FLAG** *Until effective treatment begins, patients with PVCs and serious symptoms should have continuous ECG monitoring and ambulate only with assistance.*

◆ If PVCs have a purely cardiac origin, drugs to suppress ventricular irritability may be used, such as these:
  – Amiodarone.
  – Lidocaine.
  – Procainamide.

◆ When PVCs have a noncardiac origin, treatment is aimed at correcting the cause.
  – For example, drug therapy may be adjusted or the patient's acidosis corrected.

◆ Patients who have recently developed PVCs need prompt assessment, especially if they have underlying heart disease or complex medical problems.

◆ Patients with chronic PVCs should be observed closely for the development of more frequent PVCs or more dangerous PVC patterns.

◆ If the patient is discharged on antiarrhythmic drugs, make sure family members know how to activate the emergency medical system and perform cardiopulmonary resuscitation.

Idioventricular rhythm

◆ Also known as ventricular escape rhythm.

◆ Originates in an escape pacemaker site in the ventricles.

◆ Inherent firing rate of escape pacemaker site usually 20 to 40 beats/minute.

◆ A safety mechanism because rhythm prevents ventricular standstill (asystole, the absence of electrical activity in the ventricles).

◆ Ventricular escape beats or complexes: When fewer than three QRS complexes arise from the escape pacemaker.

 LIFE-THREATENING ARRHYTHMIA

Recognizing idioventricular rhythm

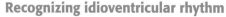

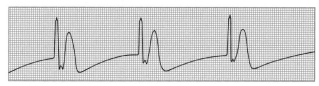

ECG characteristics

◆ Rhythm
  – Atrial: Usually can't be determined.
  – Ventricular: Usually regular.
◆ Rate
  – Atrial: Usually can't be determined.
  – Ventricular: 20 to 40 beats/ minute.
◆ P wave
  – Absent.
◆ PR interval
  – Not measurable because of absent P wave.

◆ QRS complex
  – Duration: Exceeds 0.12 second because of abnormal ventricular depolarization.
  – Configuration: Wide and bizarre.
◆ T wave
  – Abnormal.
  – Usually deflects in opposite direction from QRS complex.
◆ QT interval
  – Usually prolonged.
◆ Other
  – Commonly occurs with third-degree atrioventricular block.

◆ Accelerated idioventricular rhythm:
  – When the rate of an ectopic pacemaker site in the ventricles is less than 100 beats/minute but exceeds the inherent ventricular escape rate of 20 to 40 beats/minute.
  – Rate not fast enough to be considered VT.
  – Rhythm usually related to enhanced automaticity of ventricular tissue.
  – The same ECG characteristics as idioventricular rhythm except for heart rate.

 LIFE-THREATENING ARRHYTHMIA

Recognizing accelerated idioventricular rhythm

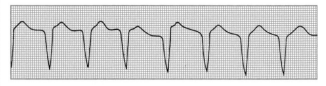

ECG characteristics

◆ Rhythm
  – Atrial: Can't be determined.
  – Ventricular: Usually regular.
◆ Rate
  – Atrial: Usually can't be determined.
  – Ventricular: 40 to 100 beats/minute.
◆ P wave
  – Absent.
  – May appear inverted after QRS complex.

◆ PR interval
  – Not measurable.
◆ QRS complex
  – Duration: Exceeds 0.12 second.
  – Configuration: Wide and bizarre.
◆ T wave
  – Abnormal.
  – Usually deflects in opposite direction from QRS complex.
◆ QT interval
  – Usually prolonged.
◆ Other
  – None.

Causes

- ◆ Digoxin toxicity.
- ◆ Drugs (beta blockers, calcium channel blockers, tricyclic anti-depressants).
- ◆ Failure of all of heart's higher pacemakers.
- ◆ Failure of supraventricular impulses to reach the ventricles because of a block in the conduction system.
- ◆ Metabolic imbalance.
- ◆ Myocardial infarction.
- ◆ Myocardial ischemia.
- ◆ Pacemaker failure.
- ◆ Sick sinus syndrome.
- ◆ Third-degree heart block.

Clinical significance

- ◆ Transient ventricular escape rhythm: Usually related to increased parasympathetic effect and not usually clinically significant.
- ◆ Continuous idioventricular rhythm: Markedly decreased cardiac output from slow ventricular rate and loss of atrial kick.

 RED FLAG *If not rapidly identified and appropriately managed, idioventricular arrhythmias can be fatal.*

Signs and symptoms

- ◆ Evidence of sharply decreased cardiac output if patient has continuous idioventricular rhythm.
- ◆ May be difficult or impossible to auscultate or palpate blood pressure.
- ◆ Possible symptoms:
  - – Dizziness.
  - – Feeling faint.
  - – Light-headedness.
  - – Loss of consciousness.

Interventions

◆ Treatment should begin immediately to increase heart rate, improve cardiac output, and establish a normal rhythm.

 RED FLAG *Treatment doesn't aim to suppress the idioventricular rhythm because this arrhythmia acts as a safety mechanism against ventricular standstill.*

◆ Atropine may be given to increase the heart rate.

 RED FLAG *Never treat an idioventricular rhythm with lidocaine or other antiarrhythmics that would suppress the escape beats.*

◆ If atropine isn't effective or the patient develops hypotension or other evidence of clinical instability, a pacemaker may be inserted to reestablish a heart rate and cardiac output sufficient to perfuse organs.

◆ A transcutaneous pacemaker may be used in an emergency until a temporary or transvenous pacemaker can be inserted.

◆ Maintain continuous ECG monitoring and constant assessment until hemodynamic stability has been restored.

◆ Keep atropine and pacemaker equipment readily available.

◆ Enforce bed rest until an effective heart rate has been maintained and the patient is stable.

◆ Tell the patient and family members about the serious nature of this arrhythmia and the treatment it requires.

◆ If the patient needs a permanent pacemaker, explain how it works, how to recognize problems, when to contact a physician, and how pacemaker function will be monitored.

Ventricular tachycardia

◆ Also called V-tach.
◆ Three or more premature ventricular contractions (PVCs) in a row with a ventricular rate above 100 beats/minute.
◆ May be monomorphic or polymorphic; sustained or non-sustained.

 LIFE-THREATENING ARRHYTHMIA

Recognizing ventricular tachycardia

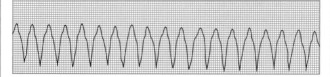

ECG characteristics

◆ Rhythm
  – Atrial: Can't be determined.
  – Ventricular: Usually regular but may be slightly irregular.
◆ Rate
  – Atrial: Can't be determined.
  – Ventricular: Usually rapid (100 to 250 beats/minute).
◆ P wave
  – Usually absent.
  – May be obscured by QRS complex.
  – Dissociated from QRS complexes.
◆ PR interval
  – Not measurable because P wave usually absent.

◆ QRS complex
  – Duration: Exceeds 0.12 second.
  – Configuration: Usually bizarre, with increased amplitude.
  – Uniform in monomorphic ventricular tachycardia (VT).
  – Constantly changes shape in polymorphic VT.
◆ T wave
  – If visible, occurs opposite the QRS complex.
◆ QT interval
  – Not measurable.
◆ Other
  – Ventricular flutter: A variation of VT.
  – Torsades de pointes: A variation of polymorphic VT, relatively rare, and sometimes difficult to distinguish from ventricular flutter.

Causes

- ◆ Usually from increased myocardial irritability, which may be triggered by:
  - – Enhanced automaticity.
  - – PVCs that occur during the downstroke of preceding T wave.
  - – Reentry in the Purkinje system.
- ◆ Other causes:
  - – Cardiomyopathy.
  - – Coronary artery disease.
  - – Drug intoxication from cocaine, procainamide, or quinidine.
  - – Electrolyte imbalance, such as hypokalemia.
  - – Heart failure.
  - – Myocardial ischemia.
  - – Myocardial infarction.
  - – Rewarming during hypothermia.
  - – Valvular heart disease.

Clinical significance

◆ Nonsustained ventricular tachycardia (VT) causes few or no symptoms.
◆ Unpredictable, with increased risk of death.
◆ May render patient hemodynamically stable with normal pulse and blood pressure, unstable with hypotension and poor peripheral pulses, or unconscious with no respirations or pulse.
◆ May deteriorate quickly to ventricular fibrillation and cardiovascular collapse because of decreased ventricular filling time and cardiac output.
◆ May lead to torsades de pointes, a variation of polymorphic VT.
◆ May be difficult to distinguish the relatively rare torsades de pointes from ventricular flutter.
◆ May be difficult to distinguish VT from supraventricular tachycardia, especially if patient has aberrant ventricular conduction.

 LIFE-THREATENING ARRHYTHMIA

Recognizing torsades de pointes

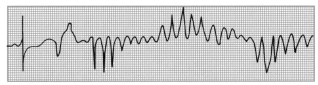

ECG characteristics

◆ Rhythm
  – Atrial: Can't be determined.
  – Ventricular: May be regular or irregular.
◆ Rate
  – Atrial: Can't be determined.
  – Ventricular: 150 to 250 beats/minute.
◆ P wave
  – Not identifiable.
  – Buried in QRS complex.
◆ PR interval
  – Not measurable because P wave can't be identified.

◆ QRS complex
  – Usually wide.
  – Usually a phasic variation in electrical polarity, with complexes that point downward for several beats, upward for several beats.
◆ T wave
  – Not discernible.
◆ QT interval
  – Prolonged.
◆ Other
  – May be paroxysmal, starting and stopping suddenly.

Signs and symptoms

◆ Possibly only minor symptoms initially.
◆ May progress quickly to cardiovascular collapse.
◆ Usually weak or absent pulses.
◆ Hypotension and decreased level of consciousness from de-creased cardiac output, quickly leading to unresponsiveness if untreated.
◆ Possible angina, heart failure, and substantial decrease in organ perfusion.

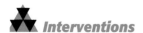

Interventions

◆ Determine whether the patient is conscious and has spontaneous respirations and a palpable carotid pulse.

 RED FLAG *Patients with pulseless VT are treated the same as those with ventricular fibrillation; they require immediate defibrillation.*

◆ If the patient is unstable, perform immediate synchronized cardioversion.

◆ If the patient is stable, folow monomorphic or polymorphic algorithm.

◆ Patient with chronic, recurrent episodes of VT unresponsive to drug therapy may need an implanted cardioverter-defibrillator (ICD).

 RED FLAG *If a patient will be discharged with an ICD or long-term antiarrhythmic therapy, make sure that family members know how to use the emergency medical system and how to perform cardiopulmonary resuscitation.*

◆ A 12-lead ECG and all other available clinical information is critical for establishing a diagnosis in a stable patient with wide QRS complexes and tachycardia of unknown type.

◆ If a definitive diagnosis of supraventricular tachycardia or VT can't be established, treatment should be guided by whether cardiac function is adequate (ejection fraction above 40%).

◆ Teach the patient and family about the serious nature of this arrhythmia and the need for prompt treatment.

Distinguishing torsades de pointes from ventricular flutter

Torsades de pointes is a variant form of ventricular tachycardia with a rapid ventricular rate that varies between 250 and 350 beats/minute. It's characterized by changing QRS complexes, with the amplitude of each successive complex gradually increasing and decreasing ("the twisting of points"). This results in an overall outline of the rhythm commonly described as *spindle-shaped.*

Ventricular flutter, although rarely recognized, results from the rapid, regular, repetitive beating of the ventricles. It's produced by a single ventricular focus firing at a rapid rate of 250 to 350 beats/minute. The hallmark of this arrhythmia is its smooth sine-wave appearance.

These illustrations show key differences in the two arrhythmias.

Torsades de pointes

◆ Spindle-shaped appearance.

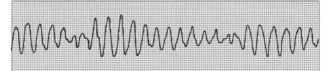

Ventricular flutter

◆ Smooth, sine-wave appearance.

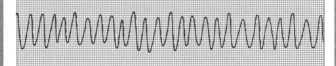

Distinguishing ventricular tachycardia from supraventricular tachycardia

Differentiating ventricular tachycardia (VT) from supraventricular tachycardia (SVT) with aberrancy is difficult. Careful assessment of a 12-lead ECG or rhythm strip can help you determine the arrhythmia with 90% accuracy.

Begin by looking at the deflection – negative or positive. Then use the following illustrations to guide your assessment. If the QRS complex is wide and mostly negative in deflection in V_1 or MCL_1, use these clues.

Ventricular tachycardia

◆ If the QRS complex has an R wave of 0.04 second or more, a slurred S (shown below, shaded), or a notched S on the downstroke (shown below at right), suspect VT.

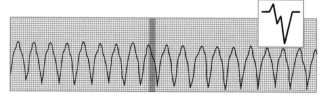

Supraventricular tachycardia

◆ If the QRS complex has an R wave of 0.04 second or more and a swift, straight S on the downstroke (shown below, shaded, and below right), suspect SVT with aberrancy.

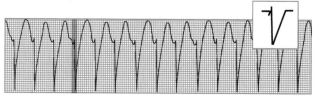

(continued)

Distinguishing ventricular tachycardia from supraventricular tachycardia *(continued)*

If the QRS complex is wide and mostly positive in deflection in V_1 or MCL_1, use these clues.

Ventricular tachycardia

◆ If the QRS complex is biphasic, suspect VT.

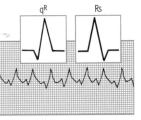

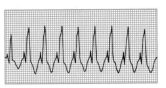

Supraventricular tachycardia

◆ If the beat is triphasic, similar to a right bundle-branch block, suspect SVT with aberrancy.

 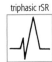

Other clues you can use if the QRS complex is wide and mostly positive in deflection in lead V$_1$ or MCL$_1$ include the following:

If the QRS complex is tall and shaped like rabbit ears, with the left peak taller than the right, suspect VT.

Taller left peak

If the QRS complex is monophasic, suspect VT.

QRS

If you still have trouble differentiating the rhythm, look at V$_6$ or MCL$_6$.

If the S wave is larger than the R wave, suspect VT.

rS

If a Q wave is present, suspect VT.

Q

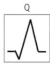

Other general criteria can also help you differentiate VT from SVT with aberrancy.

◆ A QRS complex that exceeds 0.14 second suggests VT.

◆ A regular, wide, complex rhythm suggests VT.

◆ An irregular, wide, complex rhythm suggests SVT with aberrancy.

◆ Concordant V leads (the QRS complex either mainly positive or mainly negative in all V leads) suggest VT.

◆ Atrioventricular dissociation suggests VT.

Stable monomorphic or polymorphic ventricular tachycardia algorithm

Cardioversion is an appropriate, immediate treatment for stable ventricular tachycardia (VT). Alternatives to this treatment depend on the type of VT, the patient's cardiac function, and the configuration of the QT interval. In monomorphic VT, QRS complexes keep the same form or appearance. In polymorphic VT, QRS complexes occur in more than one form, varying in appearance.

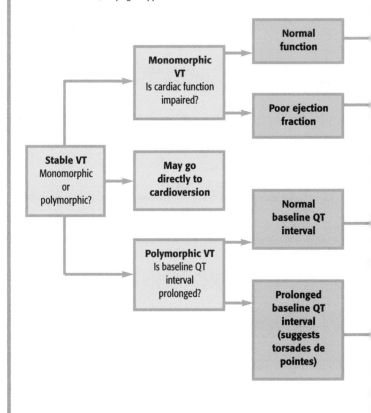

Drugs (any one)
- procainamide
- sotalol

Others acceptable
- amiodarone
- lidocaine

- amiodarone by I.V. bolus
  or
- lidocaine by I.V. push
  then
- synchronized cardioversion

Treat ischemia.

Correct electrolyte levels.

Drugs (any one)
- beta blockers
- lidocaine
- amiodarone
- procainamide
- sotalol

Cardiac function impaired

Correct abnormal electrolyte levels.

Treatment (any of these)
- magnesium
- overdrive pacing
- isoproterenol
- phenytoin
- lidocaine

Ventricular fibrillation

♦ Commonly called V-fib or VF.
♦ A chaotic, disorganized pattern of electrical activity.
♦ Electrical impulses from multiple ectopic pacemakers in the ventricles.
♦ No effective ventricular mechanical activity or contractions.
♦ No cardiac output.
♦ Untreated, the most common cause of sudden cardiac death among people not in a health care facility.

 LIFE-THREATENING ARRHYTHMIA

Recognizing ventricular fibrillation

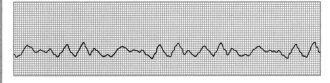

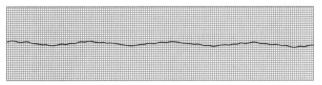

ECG characteristics

♦ Rhythm
   – Atrial: Can't be determined.
   – Ventricular: No pattern or regularity, just fibrillatory waves.
♦ Rate
   – Atrial: Can't be determined.
   – Ventricular: Can't be determined.
♦ P wave
   – Can't be determined.
♦ PR interval
   – Can't be determined.

♦ QRS complex
   – Can't be determined.
♦ T wave
   – Can't be determined.
♦ QT interval
   – Not applicable.
♦ Other
   – Electrical defibrillation more successful with coarse fibrillatory waves than with fine waves, which indicate more advanced hypoxemia and acidosis.

Causes

◆ Acid-base imbalance.
◆ Coronary artery disease.
◆ Drug toxicity, as from digoxin, procainamide, or quinidine.
◆ Electric shock.
◆ Electrolyte imbalances, such as hypercalcemia, hyperkalemia, and hypokalemia.
◆ Myocardial infarction.
◆ Myocardial ischemia.
◆ Severe hypothermia.
◆ Underlying heart disease, such as dilated cardiomyopathy.
◆ Untreated ventricular tachycardia.

Clinical significance

◆ Quivering ventricular muscle.
◆ Ineffective cardiac contractions.
◆ No cardiac output.
◆ Eventual ventricular standstill and death.

Signs and symptoms

◆ Full cardiac arrest.
◆ Unresponsive patient with no detectable blood pressure or central pulses.

 RED FLAG *Whenever you see an ECG pattern resembling VF, check the patient immediately and begin definitive treatment.*

Interventions

◆ Start prompt treatment following health care facility and emergency medical system protocols.

◆ Assess the patient to determine if the rhythm is VF.

◆ Start cardiopulmonary resuscitation (CPR).

> **RED FLAG** *CPR must be performed until the defibrillator arrives to preserve oxygen supply to the patient's brain and other vital organs.*

◆ Defibrillate the patient immediately up to three times with 200 joules, 200 to 300 joules, and then 360 joules.

◆ Give epinephrine or vasopressin if three attempts at defibrillation fail to correct the arrhythmia.

◆ Establish an airway and ventilate the patient.

◆ Consider giving such antiarrhythmics as amiodarone, lidocaine, magnesium, and procainamide.

◆ Teach the patient and family how to use the emergency medical system and an automated external defibrillator, if appropriate, following discharge from the facility.

◆ Family members may need instruction in CPR. Teach them about long-term therapies that help prevent recurrent episodes of VF, including antiarrhythmic therapy and implanted cardioverter-defibrillators.

Ventricular fibrillation and pulseless ventricular tachycardia algorithm

Ventricular fibrillation (VF) and pulseless ventricular tachycardia (VT) require aggressive, systematic treatment. Follow this algorithm for patients with these arrhythmias.

Primary ABCD survey

Focus: Basic cardiopulmonary resuscitation and defibrillation

◆ Check responsiveness.
◆ Activate emergency response system.
◆ Call for defibrillator.
◆ **A** Airway: Open the airway.
◆ **B** Breathing: Provide positive-pressure ventilations.
◆ **C** Circulation: Give chest compressions.
◆ **D** Defibrillation: Assess patient for pulseless VT and defibrillate up to three times (200 joules, 200 to 300 joules, 360 joules, or equivalent biphasic), if necessary.

↓

Rhythm after first three defibrillations?

↓

Persistent or recurrent VF or VT

Secondary ABCD survey

Focus: More advanced assessments and treatments

◆ **A** Airway: Insert airway device as soon as possible.
◆ **B** Breathing: Confirm airway device placement by examination plus confirmation device.
◆ **B** Breathing: Secure airway device (purpose-made tube holders preferred).
◆ **B** Breathing: Confirm effective oxygenation and ventilation.
◆ **C** Circulation: Establish I.V. access.
◆ **C** Circulation: Identify rhythm and monitor.
◆ **C** Circulation: Give drugs appropriate for rhythm and condition.
◆ **D** Differential diagnosis: Search for and treat reversible causes.

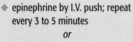

- epinephrine by I.V. push; repeat every 3 to 5 minutes
  or
- vasopressin I.V.; single dose, one time only

Resume attempts to defibrillate.

1 × 360 joules (or equivalent biphasic) within 30 to 60 seconds

Consider antiarrhythmics.
Consider buffers.

- amiodarone
- lidocaine
- magnesium
- procainamide

Resume attempts to defibrillate.

Asystole

◆ Also called ventricular asystole and ventricular standstill.
◆ Has been called the arrhythmia of death.
◆ Absence of discernible electrical activity in the ventricles.
◆ Some electrical activity possible in the atria, but no impulses conducted to the ventricles.
◆ Usually from prolonged cardiac arrest without effective resuscitation.
◆ Important to distinguish from fine ventricular fibrillation (VF), which is managed differently.

 LIFE-THREATENING ARRHYTHMIA

Recognizing asystole

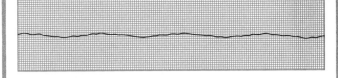

ECG characteristics

◆ Rhythm
  – Atrial: Usually indiscernible.
  – Ventricular: Not present.
◆ Rate
  – Atrial: Usually indiscernible.
  – Ventricular: Not present.
◆ P wave
  – May be present.
◆ PR interval
  – Not measurable.
◆ QRS complex
  – Absent or occasional escape beats.

◆ T wave
  – Absent.
◆ QT interval
  – Not measurable.
◆ Other
  – Looks like a nearly flat line on a rhythm strip except during chest compressions with cardiopulmonary resuscitation.
  – If patient has a pacemaker, pacer spikes may show on the strip, but no P wave or QRS complex occurs in response.

Causes

◆ Cardiac tamponade.
◆ Drug overdose.
◆ Hypothermia.
◆ Hypovolemia.
◆ Hypoxia.
◆ Massive pulmonary embolism.
◆ Myocardial infarction (coronary thrombosis).
◆ Severe electrolyte disturbances, especially hyperkalemia and hypokalemia.
◆ Severe, uncorrected acid-base disturbances, especially metabolic acidosis.
◆ Tension pneumothorax.

Clinical significance

◆ Considered a confirmation of death rather than an arrhythmia to be treated.
◆ No cardiac output or perfusion of vital organs.

 RED FLAG *Without immediate cardiopulmonary resuscitation and rapid identification and treatment of the underlying cause, asystole quickly becomes irreversible.*

Signs and symptoms

◆ The patient will be unresponsive with no spontaneous respirations, no discernible pulse, and no blood pressure.

Interventions

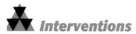 **RED FLAG** *Remember to verify asystole by checking more than one ECG lead.*

◆ Immediate treatment for asystole includes effective cardiopulmonary resuscitation, supplemental oxygen, and advanced airway control with tracheal intubation.

◆ Resuscitation should be attempted unless evidence exists that it shouldn't be performed, such as when a do-not-resuscitate order is in effect.

◆ Identify and treat potentially reversible causes.

◆ Early transcutaneous pacing may be considered, and I.V. epinephrine and atropine is given.

◆ With persistent asystole despite appropriate management, resuscitation may end.

Asystole algorithm

Few patients with asystole survive. The treatment goal is to reestablish a heart rhythm. Treatment includes pacing and appropriate medications to stimulate impulse conduction. Use the following algorithm to guide treatment of the patient with asystole.

Primary ABCD survey

Focus: Basic cardiopulmonary resuscitation and defibrillation

- Check responsiveness.
- Activate emergency response system.
- Call for defibrillator.
- **A** Airway: Open the airway.
- **B** Breathing: Provide positive-pressure ventilations.
- **C** Circulation: Give chest compressions.
- **C** Circulation: Confirm true asystole.
- **D** Defibrillation: Assess for ventricular fibrillation or pulseless ventricular tachycardia; defibrillate, if indicated.
- Rapid scene survey: Any evidence that personnel shouldn't attempt resuscitation?

Secondary ABCD survey

Focus: More advanced assessments and treatments

- **A** Airway: Insert airway device as soon as possible.
- **B** Breathing: Confirm airway device placement by examination plus confirmation device.
- **B** Breathing: Secure airway device (purpose-made tube holders preferred).
- **B** Breathing: Confirm effective oxygenation and ventilation.
- **C** Circulation: Confirm true asystole.
- **C** Circulation: Establish I.V. access.
- **C** Circulation: Identify rhythm on monitor.
- **C** Circulation: Give drugs appropriate for rhythm and condition.
- **D** Differential diagnosis: Search for and treat reversible causes.

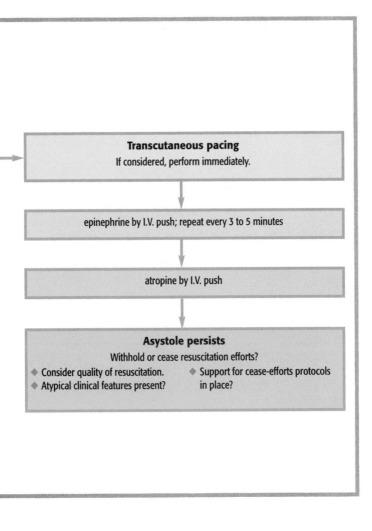

Transcutaneous pacing
If considered, perform immediately.

epinephrine by I.V. push; repeat every 3 to 5 minutes

atropine by I.V. push

Asystole persists
Withhold or cease resuscitation efforts?
◆ Consider quality of resuscitation.
◆ Atypical clinical features present?
◆ Support for cease-efforts protocols in place?

Pulseless electrical activity

◆ Some electrical activity but no detectable pulse.
◆ Electrical depolarization, but no synchronous shortening of myocardial fibers and no mechanical activity or contractions in the heart

 LIFE-THREATENING ARRHYTHMIA

Recognizing pulseless electrical activity

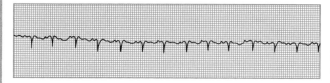

ECG characteristics

◆ Rhythm
 – Atrial: Same as underlying rhythm, becoming irregular as rate slows.
 – Ventricular: Same as underlying rhythm, becoming irregular as rate slows.
◆ Rate
 – Atrial: Reflects underlying rhythm.
 – Ventricular: Reflects underlying rhythm, eventually decreasing.
◆ P wave
 – Same as underlying rhythm, gradually flattening and then disappearing.
◆ PR interval
 – Same as underlying rhythm, eventually disappearing as P wave disappears.

◆ QRS complex
 – Same as underlying rhythm, becoming progressively wider.
◆ T wave
 – Same as underlying rhythm, eventually becoming indiscernible.
◆ QT interval
 – Same as underlying rhythm, eventually becoming indiscernible.
◆ Other
 – Usually becomes a flat line indicating asystole within several minutes.

Causes

◆ Acidosis.
◆ Cardiac tamponade.
◆ Hyperkalemia.
◆ Hypokalemia.
◆ Hypothermia.
◆ Hypovolemia.
◆ Hypoxia.
◆ Massive acute myocardial infarction.
◆ Massive pulmonary embolism.
◆ Overdoses of certain drugs, such as tricyclic antidepressants.
◆ Tension pneumothorax.

Clinical significance

- ◆ No cardiac output.
- ◆ No perfusion of vital organs.

Signs and symptoms

- ◆ Apnea and sudden loss of consciousness.
- ◆ No blood pressure.
- ◆ No pulse.

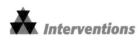 **Interventions**

♦ Start cardiopulmonary resuscitation immediately. Expect to give epinephrine and atropine according to advanced cardiac life support guidelines.

♦ Identify the cause of pulseless electrical activity and treat accordingly:
  – Volume infusion for hypovolemia from hemorrhage.
  – Pericardiocentesis for cardiac tamponade.
  – Correction of electrolyte imbalances.
  – Needle decompression or chest tube insertion for tension pneumothorax.
  – Surgery or thrombolytic therapy for massive pulmonary embolism.
  – Ventilation for hypoxemia.

♦ Pacemaker therapy is rarely effective because myocardial tissue can't respond appropriately to any electrical stimulus.

Pulseless electrical activity algorithm

After you confirm pulseless electrical activity (PEA), you need to determine its cause and treat it rapidly. Supportive measures include epinephrine and atropine.

Pulseless electrical activity

(PEA = rhythm on monitor, without detectable pulse)

Primary ABCD survey

Focus: basic cardiopulmonary resuscitation (CPR) and defibrillation
- ◆ Check responsiveness.
- ◆ Activate emergency response system.
- ◆ Call for defibrillator.
- ◆ **A** Airway: Open the airway.
- ◆ **B** Breathing: Provide positive-pressure ventilations.
- ◆ **C** Circulation: Give chest compressions.
- ◆ **D** Defibrillation: Assess for and shock ventricular fibrillation (VF) or pulseless ventricular tachycardia (VT).

Secondary ABCD survey

Focus: more advanced assessments and treatments
- ◆ **A** Airway: Insert airway device as soon as possible.
- ◆ **B** Breathing: Confirm airway device placement by examination plus confirmation device.
- ◆ **B** Breathing: Secure airway device (purpose-made tube holders are preferred).
- ◆ **B** Breathing: Confirm effective oxygenation and ventilation.
- ◆ **C** Circulation: Establish I.V. access.
- ◆ **C** Circulation: Identify rhythm and monitor.
- ◆ **C** Circulation: Give drugs appropriate for rhythm and condition.
- ◆ **C** Circulation: Assess for occult blood flow.
- ◆ **D** Differential diagnosis: Search for and treat identified reversible causes.

Review for most frequent causes.

◆ Hypovolemia
◆ Hypoxia
◆ Hydrogen ion (acidosis)
◆ Hyperkalemia or hypokalemia
◆ Hypothermia
◆ "Tablets" (drug overdose, accidents)
◆ Tamponade, cardiac
◆ Tension pneumothorax
◆ Thrombosis, coronary (acute coronary syndrome)
◆ Thrombosis, pulmonary (embolism)

epinephrine I.V. push; repeat every 3 to 5 minutes

atropine I.V.
(if PEA rate is slow);
repeat every 3 to 5 minutes as needed, to a total dose
of 0.04 mg/kg

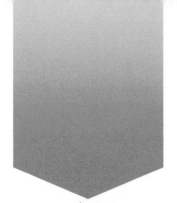

6

Atrioventricular blocks

First-degree AV block

◆ Reflects a delay in conduction of electrical impulses through the normal conduction pathway.

◆ Delayed at the level of the atrioventricular (AV) node or bundle of His.

◆ Characterized by a PR interval that exceeds 0.20 second.

Recognizing first-degree AV block

ECG characteristics

◆ Rhythm
  – Regular.
◆ Rate
  – Within normal limits.
  – Atrial the same as ventricular.
◆ P wave
  – Normal size.
  – Normal configuration.
  – Each followed by a QRS complex.
◆ PR interval
  – Prolonged.
  – More than 0.20 second (see shaded area of strip).
  – Constant.

◆ QRS complex
  – Within normal limits (0.08 second) if conduction delay occurs in atrioventricular (AV) node.
  – If more than 0.12 seconds, conduction delay may be in His-purkinje system.
◆ T wave
  – Normal size.
  – Normal configuration.
  – May be abnormal if QRS complex is prolonged.
◆ QT interval
  – Within normal limits.
◆ Other
  – None.

Causes

◆ Drugs:
  – Beta blockers.
  – Calcium channel blockers.
  – Digoxin.
◆ Myocardial infarction (MI).
◆ Myocardial ischemia.
◆ Myocarditis.
◆ Degenerative (age-related) changes in the heart.

Clinical significance

◆ May cause no symptoms in a healthy person.
◆ May be found in an otherwise normal heart.
◆ May be transient:
  – Secondary to drugs.
  – Secondary to ischemia early in an MI.
◆ May be an early sign of degenerative conduction disease.
◆ The least dangerous type of AV block.

 RED FLAG *Monitor the patient's rhythm closely. First-degree AV block may progress to a more severe type of AV block.*

Signs and symptoms

◆ Normal pulse rate.
◆ Regular rhythm.
◆ Usually no symptoms.
◆ Usually no significant effect on cardiac output.
◆ Increased interval between S_1 and S_2 on cardiac auscultation if the PR interval is extremely long.

 Interventions

◆ Identify and correct the underlying cause.
◆ Monitor the patient's electrocardiogram (ECG) to detect progression to a more serious block.
◆ Give digoxin, calcium channel blockers, and beta blockers cautiously.

Second-degree AV block type I

◆ Called Wenckebach or Mobitz I block.
◆ Each impulse from sinoatrial (SA) node delayed slightly longer than previous impulse.
◆ Pattern of progressive prolongation of PR interval.
◆ Eventually, an impulse (usually a single impulse) not conducted to ventricles.
◆ Pattern repeated after nonconducted P wave or dropped beat.

Recognizing second-degree AV block type I

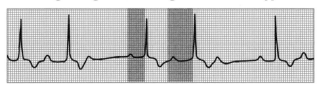

ECG characteristics

◆ Rhythm
  – Atrial: Regular.
  – Ventricular: Irregular.
◆ Rate
  – Atrial rate exceeds ventricular rate because of nonconducted beats.
  – Both rates usually within normal limits.
◆ P wave
  – Normal size.
  – Normal configuration.
  – Each followed by a QRS complex except blocked P wave.
◆ PR interval
  – Progressively longer (see shaded areas on strip) with each cycle until a P wave appears without a QRS complex.
  – Commonly described as "long, longer, dropped."
  – Slight variation in delay from cycle to cycle.

  – After the nonconducted beat, shorter than the interval preceding it.
◆ QRS complex
  – Within normal limits (0.08 second).
  – Periodically absent.
◆ T wave
  – Normal size.
  – Normal configuration.
  – Deflection may be opposite that of the QRS complex.
◆ QT interval
  – Usually within normal limits.
◆ Other
  – Wenckebach pattern of grouped beats (footprints of Wenckebach)
  – PR interval gets progressively longer and R-R interval shortens until a P wave appears without a QRS complex; cycle then repeats.

Causes

- ◆ Coronary artery disease.
- ◆ Drugs:
  - – Beta blockers.
  - – Digoxin.
  - – Calcium channel blockers.
- ◆ Increased parasympathetic tone.
- ◆ Inferior-wall MI.
- ◆ Rheumatic fever.

Clinical significance

- ◆ May occur normally in otherwise healthy person.
- ◆ Almost always transient.
- ◆ Usually resolves when underlying condition is corrected.
- ◆ May progress to a more serious form, especially if it occurs early in MI.

Signs and symptoms

- ◆ Usually no symptoms.
- ◆ Evidence of decreased cardiac output:
  - – Hypotension.
  - – Light-headedness.
- ◆ Pronounced signs and symptoms if ventricular rate is slow.

Interventions

◆ Treat only symptomatic patients.
◆ Assess tolerance for the rhythm.
◆ Assess the need to improve cardiac output.
◆ Give atropine to improve AV node conduction.

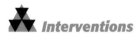 **RED FLAG** *Use atropine cautiously if the patient is having an MI. Atropine can worsen ischemia.*

◆ Teach the patient about a temporary pacemaker, if indicated.
◆ Maintain transcutaneous pacing until the arrhythmia resolves. (See *Bradycardia algorithm,* pages 38 and 39.)
◆ Evaluate patient for possible causes:
  – Drugs.
  – Myocardial ischemia.
◆ Check the ECG for more severe type of AV block.
◆ Ensure a patent I.V. line.

Second-degree AV block type II

◆ Known as Mobitz II block.
◆ Less common than type I but more serious.
◆ Occasional failure of impulses from SA node to conduct to ventricles.

Recognizing second-degree AV block type II

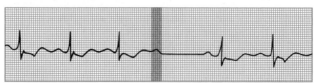

ECG characteristics

◆ Rhythm
 – Atrial: Regular.
 – Ventricular: Irregular.
 – Pauses correspond to dropped beat.
 – Irregular when block is intermittent or conduction ratio is variable.
 – Regular when conduction ratio is constant, such as 2:1 or 3:1.
◆ Rate
 – Atrial exceeds ventricular.
 – Both may be within normal limits.
◆ P wave
 – Normal size.
 – Normal configuration.
 – Some not followed by a QRS complex.
◆ PR interval
 – Usually within normal limits but may be prolonged.
 – Constant for conducted beats.
 – May be shortened after a non-conducted beat.

◆ QRS complex
 – Within normal limits or narrow if block occurs at bundle of His.
 – Widened and similar to bundle-branch block if block occurs at bundle branches.
 – Periodically absent.
◆ T wave
 – Normal size.
 – Normal configuration.
◆ QT interval
 – Within normal limits.
◆ Other
 – PR and R-R intervals don't vary before a dropped beat (see shaded area), so no warning occurs.
 – R-R interval that contains nonconducted P wave equals two normal R-R intervals.
 – Must be complete block in one bundle branch and intermittent interruption in conduction in the other bundle for a dropped beat to occur.

◆ Occurs below level of AV node at bundle of His or bundle branches (more common).
◆ Hallmarks:
  – Constant PR interval.
  – Possibly more than one nonconducted beat in succession.

Causes

◆ Anterior-wall MI.
◆ Degenerative changes in the conduction system.
◆ Organic heart disease.
◆ Severe coronary artery disease.

Clinical significance

◆ Poorer prognosis.
◆ Can lead to complete heart block.
◆ Causes low cardiac output.
◆ Symptoms are more likely to appear, particularly in these cases:
  – Slow sinus rhythm.
  – Low ratio of conducted beats to dropped beats (such as 2:1).
◆ May be difficult to distinguish from nonconducted premature atrial contractions.

Signs and symptoms

◆ Usually no symptoms with adequate cardiac output.
◆ Only occasional dropped beats with adequate cardiac output.
◆ Evidence of decreased cardiac output (as dropped beats increase):
  – Chest pain.
  – Dyspnea.
  – Fatigue.
  – Light-headedness.
◆ Hypotension.
◆ Slow pulse.
◆ Regular or irregular rhythm.

Interventions

◆ Observe the cardiac rhythm for progression to a more severe block.

◆ Evaluate the patient for correctable causes (such as ischemia).

◆ Reduce myocardial oxygen demands by keeping the patient on bed rest and giving oxygen.

◆ Teach the patient and family about pacemakers if the patient will receive one.

◆ If the patient has no serious signs and symptoms, do the following:
– Monitor the patient continuously, keeping a transcutaneous pacemaker attached to the patient or in the room.
– Prepare the patient for transvenous pacemaker insertion.

◆ If the patient has serious signs and symptoms, do the following:
– Give intravenous atropine, dopamine, epinephrine, or a combination of these drugs. (See *Bradycardia algorithm,* pages 38 and 39.)
– Use transcutaneous pacing.

 RED FLAG *Advanced cardiac life support guidelines warn that atropine can worsen ischemia during an MI. It may induce ventricular tachycardia or fibrillation if the patient has Mobitz II block and complete heart block.*

Distinguishing second-degree AV block type II from nonconducted PACs

An isolated nonconducted P wave (a P wave not followed by a QRS complex, as shown in the shaded areas below) may result from second-degree atrioventricular (AV) block type II or a nonconducted premature atrial contraction (PAC). Thinking a patient has nonconducted PACs when he really has AV block can have serious consequences. The former is usually benign, but the latter can be life-threatening.

Second-degree AV block type II

If the P-P interval is constant, including the extra P wave, it's second-degree AV block type II.

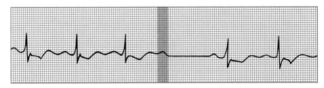

Nonconducted PAC

If the P-P interval, including the extra P wave, isn't constant, it's a nonconducted PAC.

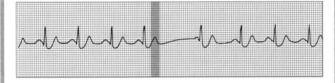

Third-degree AV block

◆ Called complete heart block or AV dissociation.
◆ Complete absence of impulse conduction between atria and ventricles.
◆ Variable treatment and prognosis depending on anatomic level of block.

Recognizing third-degree AV block

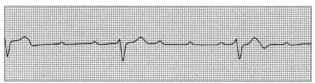

ECG characteristics

◆ Rate
  – Atrial: 60 to 100 beats/minute (atria act independently under control of sinoatrial node).
  – Ventricular: Usually 40 to 60 beats/minute in intranodal block (a junctional escape rhythm).
  – Ventricular: Usually less than 40 beats/minute in infranodal block (a ventricular escape rhythm).
◆ P wave
  – Normal size.
  – Normal configuration.
  – May be buried in QRS complexes or T waves.
◆ PR interval
  – Not measurable.
◆ QRS complex
  – Configuration depends on location of escape mechanism and origin of ventricular depolarization.

– Appears normal if block at the level of atrioventricular (AV) node or bundle of His.
– Widened if block at the level of bundle branches.
◆ T wave
  – Normal size.
  – Normal configuration.
  – May be abnormal if QRS complex originates in ventricle.
◆ QT interval
  – Within normal limits.
◆ Other
  – Atria and ventricles depolarized from different pacemakers and beat independently of each other (AV dissociation).
  – P waves occur without QRS complexes.

Causes

- ◆ At anatomic level of AV node:
  - – AV node damage.
  - – Increased parasympathetic tone.
  - – Inferior-wall MI.
  - – Toxic effects of drugs (digoxin, propranolol).
- ◆ At infranodal level:
  - – Extensive anterior MI.

Clinical significance

- ◆ At AV node, with a junctional escape rhythm:
  - – Usually transient.
  - – Usually favorable prognosis.
- ◆ At infranodal level:
  - – Unstable pacemaker.
  - – Common episodes of ventricular asystole.
  - – Less favorable prognosis.
  - – Life-threatening because of slow ventricular rate and significantly decreased cardiac output.
- ◆ Decreased cardiac output from loss of AV synchrony and resulting loss of atrial kick.
- ◆ Severity depends on:
  - – Ventricular rate.
  - – Patient's ability to compensate for decreased cardiac output.

Signs and symptoms

◆ A few patients relatively free of symptoms except for exercise intolerance, unexplained fatigue.
◆ Changes in level of consciousness.
◆ Changes in mental status.
◆ Chest pain.
◆ Diaphoresis.
◆ Dyspnea.
◆ Hypotension.
◆ Light-headedness.
◆ Pallor.
◆ Severe fatigue.
◆ Slow peripheral pulse rate.

 Interventions

◆ Make sure patient has a patent I.V. line.
◆ Give oxygen.
◆ Assess patient for correctable causes of arrhythmia (such as drugs, myocardial ischemia).
◆ Minimize patient's activity level.
◆ Maintain bed rest.
◆ If the patient has serious signs and symptoms, provide immediate treatment that includes doing the following:
– Maintain transcutaneous pacing (most effective).
– Give I.V. atropine, dopamine, epinephrine, or a combination (for short-term use in emergencies).

 RED FLAG *Atropine isn't indicated for third-degree AV block with wide-complex ventricular escape beats.*

◆ If the patient has no symptoms, maintain temporary transvenous pacing until the need for a permanent pacemaker is determined.

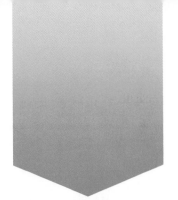

7

ECG effects of
electrolyte imbalances

Hyperkalemia

◆ Serum potassium level above 5.0 mEq/L.

ECG effects of hyperkalemia

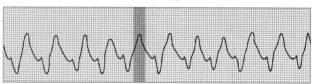

ECG characteristics

◆ Rhythm
  – Regular.
◆ Rate
  – Within normal limits.
◆ P wave
  – Low amplitude in mild hyper-
    kalemia.
  – Wide and flattened in moderate
    hyperkalemia.
  – Not discernible in severe hyper-
    kalemia.
◆ PR interval
  – Normal or prolonged.
  – Not measurable if P wave can't
    be detected.

◆ QRS complex
  – Widened.
◆ T wave
  – Tall and peaked (the key finding,
    as shown in shaded area).
◆ QT interval
  – Shortened.
◆ Other
  – Intraventricular conduction dis-
    turbances common.
  – ST segment may be elevated in
    severe hyperkalemia.

Causes

◆ Increased potassium intake:
  – Dietary.
  – I.V. administration of penicillin G, potassium supplements, or banked whole blood.
◆ A shift of potassium from intracellular to extracellular fluid with changes in cell membrane permeability or damage:
  – Acidosis.
  – Burns.
  – Cell hypoxia.
  – Extensive surgery.
  – Insulin deficiency.
  – Massive crush injuries.
◆ Decreased renal excretion:
  – Addison's disease.
  – Decreased production and secretion of aldosterone.
  – Renal failure.
  – Use of potassium-sparing diuretics.

Clinical significance

◆ With increased extracellular potassium level and no significant change in intracellular potassium level:
  – Cell becomes less negative (partially depolarized).
  – Resting cell membrane potential decreases.
◆ With mild increase in extracellular potassium level:
  – Cells repolarize faster.
  – Cells become more irritable.
◆ With critical increase in extracellular potassium level:
  – Cells can't repolarize.
  – Cells can't respond to electrical stimuli.

 RED FLAG *When cells can't repolarize or respond to electrical stimuli, the patient may develop cardiac standstill or asystole.*

Signs and symptoms

♦ Mild hyperkalemia:
  - Diarrhea.
  - Intestinal cramping.
  - Neuromuscular irritability.
  - Restlessness.
  - Tingling lips and fingers.
♦ Severe hyperkalemia:
  - Loss of muscle tone.
  - Muscle weakness.
  - Paralysis.

 Interventions

♦ Appropriate interventions vary:
  - Severity of hyperkalemia.
  - Patient's signs and symptoms.
♦ Identify underlying cause.
♦ Give I.V. calcium gluconate to decrease neuromuscular irritability.
♦ Give I.V. insulin to facilitate entry of potassium into cells.

 RED FLAG *When giving insulin for hyperkalemia, keep the patient from becoming hypoglycemic by giving I.V. dextrose at the same time.*

♦ Give I.V. sodium bicarbonate to correct metabolic acidosis.
♦ Give oral or rectal cation exchange resins (sodium polystyrene sulfonate) that exchange sodium for potassium in the intestine.
♦ Provide dialysis:
  - May be needed with renal failure or severe hyperkalemia.
  - Removes excess potassium.
♦ Monitor serum potassium levels closely.
♦ Identify and manage arrhythmias.

Hypokalemia

◆ Potassium level below 3.5 mEq/L.

ECG effects of hypokalemia

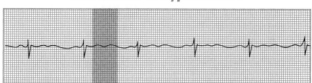

ECG characteristics

◆ Rhythm
  – Regular.
◆ Rate
  – Within normal limits.
◆ P wave
  – Normal size.
  – Normal configuration.
  – May be peaked in severe hypokalemia.
◆ PR interval
  – May be prolonged.
◆ QRS complex
  – Within normal limits.
  – Possibly widened.
  – Prolonged in severe hypokalemia.

◆ T wave
  – Decreased amplitude.
  – Becomes flat as potassium level drops, and U wave appears (the key finding, as shown in shaded area).
  – Flattens completely in severe hypokalemia and may become inverted.
  – May fuse with increasingly prominent U wave.
◆ QT interval
  – Usually indiscernible as T wave flattens.
◆ Other
  – Depressed ST segment.
  – Increased amplitude and prominence of U wave as hypokalemia worsens; may fuse with T wave.

Causes

◆ GI disorders:
  – Continuous nasogastric drainage.
  – Diarrhea.
  – Drainage tubes.
  – Intestinal fistulae.
  – Laxative abuse.
  – Vomiting.
◆ Renal disorders:
  – Increased secretion of potassium by the distal tubule.
◆ Low serum magnesium level
◆ Excessive aldosterone secretion
◆ Drugs:
  – Antibiotics, such as amphotericin B or gentamicin.
  – Diuretics.
◆ Increased entry of potassium into cells:
  – Alkalosis, especially respiratory.
  – Catecholamines.
◆ Reduced potassium intake or dietary deficiency.

Clinical significance

◆ If extracellular potassium level decreases rapidly and intracellular potassium level doesn't change:
  – Resting membrane potential becomes more negative.
  – Cell membrane becomes hyperpolarized.
  – Cardiac effects result.
◆ Possibly dangerous ventricular arrhythmias:
  – Ventricular repolarization is delayed because potassium contributes that phase of the action potential.
◆ Increased risk of digoxin toxicity.

 RED FLAG *Hypokalemia may result in digoxin toxicity. Monitor serum digoxin and potassium levels closely at the start of therapy and until maintenance doses are determined.*

Signs and symptoms

◆ Smooth muscle atony:
  – Anorexia.
  – Constipation.
  – Intestinal distention.
  – Paralytic ileus.
  – Nausea.
  – Vomiting.
◆ Skeletal muscle weakness:
  – First in larger muscles of arms and legs.
  – Eventually in the diaphragm, causing respiratory arrest.

 RED FLAG *Monitor the patient closely for early evidence of skeletal muscle weakness because it may progress to respiratory arrest.*

◆ Cardiac arrhythmias:
  – Atrioventricular (AV) block.
  – Bradycardia.
  – Ventricular arrhythmias.

 Interventions

◆ Identify and correct underlying causes.
◆ Correct acid-base imbalances.
◆ Replace potassium losses.
◆ Prevent further losses.
◆ Encourage intake of potassium-rich foods and fluids.
◆ Give oral or I.V. potassium supplements.
◆ Monitor serum potassium levels closely.
◆ Identify and manage cardiac arrhythmias.

Hypercalcemia

◆ Serum calcium level above 10.5 mg/dl.

ECG effects of hypercalcemia

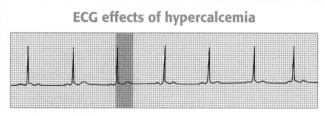

ECG characteristics

◆ Rhythm
  – Regular.
◆ Rate
  – Within normal limits.
  – Possible bradycardia.
◆ P wave
  – Normal size.
  – Normal configuration.
◆ PR interval
  – May be prolonged.
◆ QRS complex
  – Within normal limits.
  – May be prolonged.

◆ T wave
  – Normal size.
  – Normal configuration.
  – May be depressed.
◆ QT interval
  – Shortened from increased calcium level (the key finding, as shown in shaded area).
◆ Other
  – Shortened ST segment.

Causes

◆ Excess vitamin D intake.
◆ Bone metastasis and calcium resorption from cancers of the breast, prostate, or cervix.
◆ Hyperparathyroidism.
◆ Sarcoidosis.
◆ Parathyroid hormone (PTH)–producing tumors.

Clinical significance

◆ Cell membrane becomes refractory to depolarization.
◆ Loss of cell membrane excitability causes cardiac symptoms.
◆ Ventricular depolarization and repolarization are accelerated.
◆ Bradyarrhythmias and varying degrees of AV block may occur.

Signs and symptoms

◆ Anorexia.
◆ Behavioral changes.
◆ Constipation.
◆ Fatigue.
◆ Impaired renal function.
◆ Lethargy.
◆ Nausea.
◆ Reciprocal decrease in serum phosphate levels.
◆ Renal calculi (precipitates of Ca^{++} salts).
◆ Weakness.

 Interventions

◆ Identify and manage the underlying cause.
◆ Use the severity of the patient's symptoms to guide treatment.
◆ Give oral phosphate as long as renal function is normal.
◆ Give large volumes of I.V. normal saline solution to enhance renal excretion of calcium.
◆ Give corticosteroids and calcitonin. Patients with renal failure receive dialysis.

Hypocalcemia

◆ Serum calcium level below 8.5 mg/dl.

ECG effects of hypocalcemia

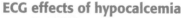

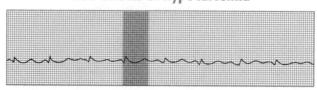

ECG characteristics

◆ Rhythm
 – Regular.
◆ Rate
 – Within normal limits.
◆ P wave
 – Normal size.
 – Normal configuration.
◆ PR interval
 – Within normal limits.
◆ QRS complex
 – Within normal limits.

◆ T wave
 – Normal size.
 – Normal configuration.
 – May be flat or inverted.
◆ QT interval
 – Prolonged from decreased calcium level (the key finding, as shown in shaded area).
◆ Other
 – Prolonged ST segment.

Causes

- ◆ Inadequate calcium intake:
  - – Green, leafy vegetables.
  - – Dairy products.
- ◆ Excessive phosphorus intake:
  - – Binds with calcium.
  - – Prevents calcium absorption.
- ◆ Blood administration:
  - – Citrate solution in stored blood binds with calcium.
- ◆ Pancreatitis:
  - – Decreases ionized calcium.
- ◆ Neoplastic bone metastases:
  - – Decrease serum calcium levels.
- ◆ Vitamin D deficiency:
  - – Inadequate intake.
  - – Inadequate exposure to sunlight.
- ◆ Malabsorption of fats.
- ◆ Decreased PTH:
  - – Removal of parathyroid glands.
- ◆ Metabolic or respiratory alkalosis.
- ◆ Hypoalbuminemia.

Clinical significance

- ◆ Increased neuromuscular excitability.
- ◆ Characteristic ECG changes from:
  - – Prolonged ventricular depolarization.
  - – Decreased cardiac contractility.

Signs and symptoms

◆ Carpopedal spasm.
◆ Circumoral and digital paresthesias.
◆ Confusion.
◆ Hyperactive bowel sounds.
◆ Hyperreflexia.
◆ Intestinal cramping.
◆ Positive Chvostek's sign.
◆ Positive Trousseau's sign.

 RED FLAG *Keep calcium gluconate on hand for a patient with a positive Trousseau's or Chvostek's sign. Hypocalcemia may progress quickly to tetany, seizures, respiratory arrest, and death.*

◆ Severe hypoclacemia:
  – Tetany.
  – Seizures.
  – Respiratory arrest.
  – Death.

 Interventions

◆ Identify and manage underlying causes.
◆ Monitor serum calcium levels.
◆ Give I.V. calcium gluconate for severe symptoms.
◆ Replace calcium orally.
◆ Identify and manage cardiac arrhythmias.
◆ Instruct the patient to decrease phosphate intake.

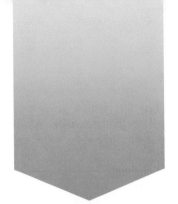

8

ECG effects of antiarrhythmics

Class I antiarrhythmics

♦ Known as sodium channel blockers or fast channel blockers.
♦ Block sodium influx during phase 0 of action potential.
♦ Subdivided into three groups (classes IA, IB, and IC) based on drug effects:
   – Interactions with cardiac sodium channels.
   – Effects on duration of action potential.

Class IA antiarrhythmics

♦ Examples:
   – Disopyramide.
   – Procainamide.
   – Quinidine.
♦ Have intermediate interaction with sodium channels.
♦ Cardiac effects:
   – Lengthen duration of action potential.
   – Depress rate of depolarization.

ECG effects of class IA antiarrhythmics

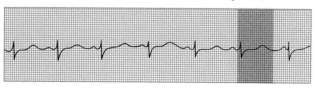

ECG characteristics

♦ Rhythm
   – No change in underlying rhythm.
♦ Rate
   – No change.
♦ P wave
   – No change.
♦ PR interval
   – No change.
♦ QRS complex
   – Slightly widened.
   – Increased widening: An early sign of toxicity.

♦ T wave
   – May be flattened or inverted.
♦ QT interval
   – Prolonged (see shaded area of strip), increasing the probability of polymorphic ventricular tachycardia.
♦ Other
   – Possible U wave.

– Prolong repolarization.
– Lengthen refractory period.
– Reduce conductivity.

Class IB antiarrhythmics

◆ Examples:
  – Lidocaine.
  – Mexiletine.
  – Phenytoin.
  – Tocainide.
◆ Interact rapidly with sodium channels.
◆ May block sodium influx during phase 0, which depresses rate of depolarization.
◆ Cardiac effects:
  – Slow phase 0 of the action potential.
  – Shorten phase 3 of the action potential.
  – May shorten repolarization and duration of action potential.
  – Suppress ventricular ectopy.
  – May suppress ventricular automaticity in ischemic tissue.
  – May affect QRS complex.

ECG effects of class IB antiarrhythmics

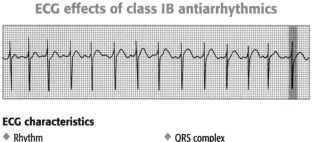

ECG characteristics

◆ Rhythm
  – No change in underlying rhythm.
◆ Rate
  – No change.
◆ P wave
  – No change.
◆ PR interval
  – May be slightly shortened.

◆ QRS complex
  – Slightly widened, as shown in shaded area.
◆ T wave
  – No change.
◆ QT interval
  – Shortened.
◆ Other
  – None.

Class IC antiarrhythmics

◆ Examples:
  – Flecainide.
  – Propafenone.
  – Moricizine (shares properties of classes IA, IB, and IC).
◆ Block sodium influx during phase 0, which depresses the rate of depolarization
◆ Interact slowly with sodium channels.
◆ Cardiac effects:
  – May have no effect on action potential duration or may minimally increase it.
  – Slow phase 0 of action potential.
  – Decrease conduction.
  – No effect on repolarization.

 RED FLAG *Class IC antiarrhythmics are usually reserved for refractory arrhythmias because they may cause or worsen arrhythmias.*

ECG effects of class IC antiarrhythmics

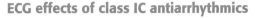
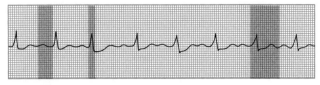

ECG characteristics

◆ Rhythm
  – No change in underlying rhythm.
◆ Rate
  – No change.
◆ P wave
  – No change.
◆ PR interval
  – Prolonged, as shown in shaded area at left of strip.

◆ QRS complex
  – Widened, as shown in shaded area in center of strip.
◆ T wave
  – No change.
◆ QT interval
  – Prolonged, as shown in shaded area at right of strip.
◆ Other
  – None.

Class II antiarrhythmics

◆ Known as beta blockers. Examples:
  – Acebutolol.
  – Esmolol.
  – Propranolol.
◆ Block beta receptors in sympathetic nervous system.
◆ Inhibit sympathetic activity.
◆ Cardiac effects:
  – Diminish phase 4 depolarization.
  – Shorten duration of action potential.
  – Depress automaticity of sinoatrial (SA) node.
  – Increase refractory period of atrial and atrioventricular (AV) junctional tissues, which slows conduction.
◆ Treat supraventricular and ventricular arrhythmias, especially those caused by excess circulating catecholamines.
◆ Cardioselective beta blockers:
  – Block only beta$_1$ receptors.
◆ Noncardioselective beta blockers:
  – May block beta$_1$ and beta$_2$ receptors.
  – May cause vasoconstriction.
  – May cause bronchospasm.

 RED FLAG *Use class II antiarrhythmics cautiously in patients with pulmonary disease.*

ECG effects of class II antiarrhythmics

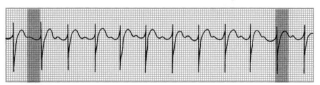

ECG characteristics

♦ Rhythm
 – No change in underlying rhythm.
♦ Rate
 – Atrial: Decreased.
 – Ventricular: Decreased.
♦ P wave
 – No change.
♦ PR interval
 – Slightly prolonged, as shown in shaded area at left of strip.

♦ QRS complex
 – No change.
♦ T wave
 – No change.
♦ QT interval
 – Slightly shortened, as shown in shaded area at right of strip.
♦ Other
 – None.

Class III antiarrhythmics

◆ Known as potassium channel blockers. Examples:
  – Amiodarone.
  – Dofetilide.
  – Ibutilide.
  – Sotalol (a nonselective beta blocker with mainly Class III properties).
◆ Cardiac effects:
  – Increase duration of action potential and effective refractory period.
  – Block movement of potassium during phase 3 of the action potential.
  – Prolong the effective refractory period.

ECG effects of class III antiarrhythmics

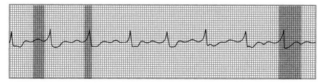

ECG characteristics

◆ Rhythm
  – No change.
◆ Rate
  – No change.
◆ P wave
  – No change.
◆ PR interval
  – Prolonged, as shown in shaded area at left.

◆ QRS complex
  – Widened, as shown in shaded area at center.
◆ T wave
  – No change.
◆ QT interval
  – Prolonged, as shown in shaded area at right.
◆ Other
  – None.

Class IV antiarrhythmics

◆ Known as calcium channel blockers or slow channel blockers. Examples:
- Diltiazem.
- Verapamil.
◆ Cardiac effects:
- Block movement of calcium during phase 2 of the action potential.
- Slow conduction.
- Increase refractory period of calcium-dependent tissues, including the AV node.
- Decrease contractility.

ECG effects of class IV antiarrhythmics

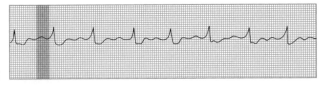

ECG characteristics

◆ Rhythm
- No change.
◆ Rate
- Atrial: Decreased.
- Ventricular: Decreased.
◆ P wave
- No change.
◆ PR interval
- Prolonged, as shown in shaded area.

◆ QRS complex
- No change.
◆ T wave
- No change.
◆ QT interval
- No change.
◆ Other
- None.

Digoxin

◆ Most commonly used cardiac glycoside.
◆ Inhibits adenosine triphosphatase.
 – An enzyme found in plasma membrane.
 – Acts as a pump to exchange sodium ions for potassium ions.
 – Enhances movement of calcium from extracellular space to intracellular space.
 – Strengthens myocardial contractions.
◆ Exerts direct effects on electrical properties of the heart.
 – Shortens action potential.
 – Shortens atrial and ventricular refractoriness.
◆ Exerts autonomic effects on electrical properties of the heart.
 – Involves sympathetic and parasympathetic systems.
 – Enhances vagal tone.
 – Slows conduction through the SA and AV nodes.
◆ Used to treat heart failure.
◆ Used to treat certain arrhythmias:
 – Paroxysmal supraventricular tachycardia.
 – Atrial fibrillation.
 – Atrial flutter.
◆ Has a very narrow range of therapeutic effectiveness.
◆ May produce toxic levels.

 RED FLAG *At toxic levels, digoxin may cause numerous arrhythmias, including paroxysmal atrial tachycardia with block, AV block, atrial and junctional tachyarrhythmias, and ventricular arrhythmias.*

ECG effects of digoxin

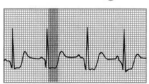

ECG characteristics

◆ Rhythm
  – No change.
◆ Rate
  – Atrial: Decreased.
  – Ventricular: Decreased.
◆ P wave
  – May be notched.
◆ PR interval
  – Shortened.
◆ QRS complex
  – No change.
◆ T wave
  – Decreased amplitude.

◆ QT interval
  – Shortened because of shortened ST segment.
◆ Other
  – Characteristic sagging (scooping or sloping) of ST segment.
  – ST segment depressed in opposite direction of QRS deflection, as shown in shaded area.
  – Shortened ST segment.

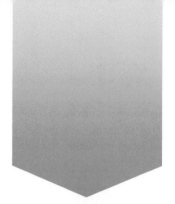

9

Pacemakers and implantable cardioverter-defibrillators

- A pacemaker is a device that stimulates the myocardium to depolarize by generating electrical impulses and conducting them to the heart.
- Typically, a pacemaker may be needed after a myocardial infarction (MI) or cardiac surgery. Pacemakers are commonly used to treat irreversible heart conduction problems, and they may be used for other indications as well:
  - Atrioventricular (AV) block.
  - Symptomatic bradycardia.
  - Sinus node dysfunction.
  - Arrhythmia suppression (long QT interval).
  - Treatment of drug-induced bradycardia.
  - Improvement of exercise capacity with rate response.
  - Cardiac resynchronization (biventricular pacing for congestive heart failure).
- An implantable cardioverter-defibrillator is used mainly for life-threatening arrhythmias.

Pacemaker components

◆ A pacemaker has three main components: A pulse generator, pacing leads or wires, and one or more electrodes at the distal ends of leadwires.

Pulse generator

◆ The generator contains a power source (battery) and electronic circuitry.

◆ It creates an electrical impulse that moves through the pacing leads to the electrodes, transmitting that impulse to the heart muscle and causing the heart to depolarize.

◆ Typically, the battery contains lithium iodide and can last 5 to 10 years depending on the frequency of pacing.

◆ Sensing, output, and timing circuits determine how the pacemaker responds to the heart's electrical activity.

◆ A microprocessor (computer chip with memory) can increase the pacemaker's capabilities and data storage.

◆ Telemetry can be used to allow communication between the pulse generator and an external programmer for reprogramming and data retrieval.

Leads and electrodes

- Leads consist of insulated conductors (low-voltage wires) and electrodes.
- Electrodes sense the heart's electrical activity.
- Leads carry information from the electrodes to the pulse generator and electrical impulses from the generator to the heart muscle.
- In single-chamber pacing, a lead is placed in an atrium or a ventricle.
- In dual-chamber or AV pacing, leads are placed in both an atrium and a ventricle.

Pacing leads

Pacing leads have either one electrode (unipolar) or two (bipolar). These illustrations show the difference between the two leads.

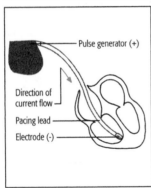

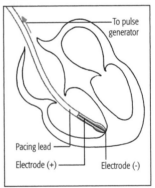

Unipolar lead

In a unipolar system, electrical current moves from the pulse generator through the leadwire to the negative pole. From there, it stimulates the heart and returns to the pulse generator's metal surface (the positive pole) to complete the circuit.

Bipolar lead

In a bipolar system, current flows from the pulse generator through the leadwire to the negative pole at the tip. At that point, it stimulates the heart and then flows back to the positive pole to complete the circuit.

ECG effects of pacemakers

- The most prominent electrocardiogram (ECG) characteristic produced by a pacemaker is known as a pacemaker spike.
- The spike occurs when the pacemaker sends an electrical impulse to the heart muscle.
- It appears as a vertical line on the ECG tracing.

Pacemaker spikes

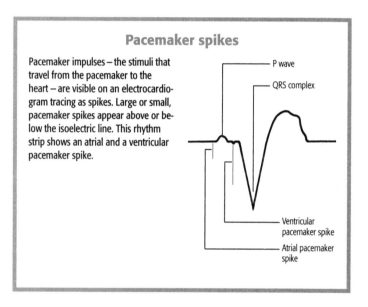

Pacemaker impulses – the stimuli that travel from the pacemaker to the heart – are visible on an electrocardiogram tracing as spikes. Large or small, pacemaker spikes appear above or below the isoelectric line. This rhythm strip shows an atrial and a ventricular pacemaker spike.

P wave

QRS complex

Ventricular pacemaker spike

Atrial pacemaker spike

◆ Collectively, a group of spikes is called pacemaker artifact.
◆ When the pacemaker simulates the atria, it causes certain effects:
  – The spike is followed by a P wave, the patient's baseline QRS, and a T wave.
  – This pattern represents successful pacing (known as capture) of the myocardium.
  – The P wave may appear different from the patient's normal P wave.
◆ When the pacemaker stimulates the ventricles, it causes certain effects:
  – The spike is followed by a QRS complex and a T wave.
  – The QRS complex appears wider than the patient's own QRS complex because of the way the pacemaker depolarizes the ventricles.
◆ When the pacemaker stimulates both the atria and ventricles, it causes certain effects:
  – The spike is followed by a P wave, and then a spike, and then a QRS complex.

Pacemaker codes

◆ A code, usually three or four letters long, is commonly used to describe pacemaker mode or function.

Pacemaker coding systems

The capabilities of permanent pacemakers can be described by a five-letter coding system. Typically, only the first three letters are used.

First letter

The first letter identifies which heart chambers are paced:
◆ V = Ventricle.
◆ A = Atrium.
◆ D = Dual – ventricle and atrium.
◆ 0 = None.

Second letter

The second letter signifies the heart chamber where the pacemaker senses intrinsic activity:
◆ V = Ventricle.
◆ A = Atrium.
◆ D = Dual.
◆ 0 = None.

Third letter

The third letter indicates the pacemaker's mode of response to the intrinsic electrical activity it senses in the atrium or ventricle:
◆ T = Triggers pacing.
◆ I = Inhibits pacing.
◆ D = Dual – can be triggered or inhibited depending on the mode and where intrinsic activity occurs.
◆ 0 = None – doesn't change mode in response to sensed activity.

Fourth letter

The fourth letter describes the degree of programmability and the presence or absence of an adaptive rate response:
◆ P = Basic functions programmable.
◆ M = Multiprogrammable parameters.
◆ C = Communicating functions, such as telemetry.
◆ R = Rate responsiveness – rate adjusts to fit the patient's metabolic needs and achieve normal hemodynamic status.
◆ 0 = None.

Fifth letter

The fifth letter denotes the pacemaker's response to a tachyarrhythmia:
◆ P = Pacing ability – the pacemaker's rapid burst paces the heart at a rate above its intrinsic rate to override the tachycardia source.
◆ S = Shock – an implantable cardioverter-defibrillator identifies ventricular tachycardia and delivers a shock to stop the arrhythmia.
◆ D = Dual ability to shock and pace.
◆ 0 = None.

Pacing modes

◆ The pacing mode refers to the programming and capabilities of the particular device.

◆ A mode is selected based on the status of the patient's intrinsic heart rhythm and the indication for pacing.

AAI and VVI pacemakers

AAI and VVI pacemakers are single-chamber pacemakers. The electrode is placed in the atrium for an AAI pacemaker, in the ventricle for a VVI pacemaker. These rhythm strips show how each pacemaker works.

AAI pacemaker

An AAI pacemaker senses and paces only the atria. As shown in the shaded area below, a P wave follows each atrial spike (atrial depolarization).The QRS complexes reflect the heart's own conduction.

This pacemaker requires a functioning atrioventricular node and intact conduction system. It may be used in patients who have symptomatic sinus bradycardia or sick sinus syndrome.

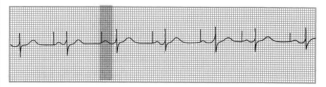

VVI pacemaker

A VVI pacemaker senses and paces the ventricles. When each spike is followed by a QRS complex (depolarization), as shown here, the rhythm is said to reflect 100% capture.

This pacemaker may be used in patients who have chronic atrial fibrillation with slow ventricular response and those who need infrequent pacing.

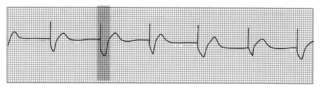

DVI and DDD pacemakers

DVI pacemaker

A committed DVI pacemaker (also known as an AV sequential pacemaker) senses ventricular activity and paces the atria and ventricles, firing despite the intrinsic QRS complex. The rhythm strip below shows the effects of a committed DVI pacemaker. Notice that in two of the complexes, shown with shaded areas, the pacemaker didn't sense the intrinsic QRS complex because the complex occurred during the AV interval, when the pacemaker was already committed to fire.

With a noncommitted DVI pacemaker, spikes wouldn't appear after the QRS complex because the stimulus to pace the ventricles would be inhibited. This pacemaker is used in patients with AV block or sick sinus syndrome.

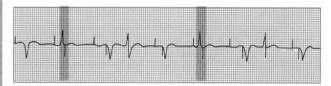

DDD pacemaker

A dual chamber pacemaker (with one lead in the atrium and another in the ventricle) provides versatile programming functions and can sense and pace in both the atrium and ventricle. This type of pacemaker mimics the normal cardiac cycle and maintains atrioventricular (AV) synchrony. It may be used for patients with chronic or intermittent AV block and for those who need atrial pacing or have delayed AV conduction or an increased risk of heart block.

When evaluating the rhythm strip of a patient with a DDD pacemaker, keep several points in mind.

♦ If the patient has an adequate intrinsic rhythm, the pacemaker won't fire; it doesn't need to.

♦ If you see an intrinsic P wave followed by a ventricular pacemaker spike, the pacemaker is tracking the atrial rate and assuring a ventricular response.

♦ If you see a pacemaker spike before a P wave, followed by an intrinsic ventricular QRS complex, the atrial rate is falling below the lower rate limit, causing the atrial channel to fire. Normal conduction to the ventricles follows.

♦ If you see a pacemaker spike before a P wave and before the QRS complex, no intrinsic activity is taking place in either the atria or ventricles.

(continued)

DVI and DDD pacemakers *(continued)*

This rhythm strip shows the effects of a DDD pacemaker. Complexes 1, 2, 4, and 7 show the atrial-synchronous mode, set at a rate of 70. The patient has an intrinsic P wave, so the pacemaker only ensures that the ventricles respond. Complexes 3, 5, 8, 10, and 12 are intrinsic ventricular depolarizations. The pacemaker senses them and doesn't fire. In complexes 6, 9, and 11, the pacemaker is pacing the atria and ventricles in sequence. In complex 13, only the atria are paced; the ventricles respond on their own.

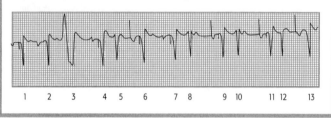

Asynchronous pacing modes

◆ Examples include AOO, VOO, and DOO.
◆ No sensing is involved; the pacemaker paces regardless of intrinsic impulses.
◆ The system provides pacing at a lower, programmed rate.
◆ Usually this approach is used temporarily in pacemaker-dependent patients to ensure pacing during certain surgical and diagnostic procedures.

Types of pacemakers

◆ A pacemaker may be permanent or temporary.
◆ Temporary pacemakers may be transvenous, epicardial, transcutaneous, or transthoracic.
◆ Certain pacemakers pace both the left and right ventricles.

Permanent pacemaker

◆ A pacemaker may be implanted permanently when a patient has an arrhythmia, commonly one of these:
  – Symptomatic bradyarrhythmia.
  – Tachyarrhythmia.
  – Sick sinus syndrome.
  – Varying degrees of AV block.

Placing a permanent pacemaker

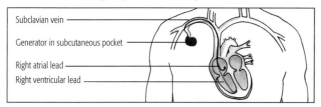

Subclavian vein
Generator in subcutaneous pocket
Right atrial lead
Right ventricular lead

Implanting a pacemaker is a simple surgical procedure performed with local anesthesia and conscious sedation. To implant an endocardial pacemaker, the surgeon usually selects a transvenous route and begins lead placement by inserting a catheter percutaneously or by venous cutdown. Then, using fluoroscopic guidance, the surgeon threads the catheter through the vein until the tip reaches the endocardium.

Lead placement

For lead placement in the atrium, the tip must lodge in the right atrium or coronary sinus, as shown here. For placement in the ventricle, it must lodge in the right ventricular apex in one of the interior muscular ridges, or trabeculae.

Implanting the generator

When the lead is in proper position, the surgeon secures the pulse generator in a subcutaneous pocket of tissue just below the patient's clavicle. Changing the generator's battery or microchip circuitry requires only a shallow incision over the site and a quick exchange of components.

BIVENTRICULAR PACEMAKER

- ◆ Also referred to as cardiac resynchronization therapy. Used to treat patients with moderate to severe heart failure who have left ventricular dysynchrony.
- ◆ Uses traditional pacing leads in right atrium and ventricle.
- ◆ Adds a pacing lead for the left ventricle and additional pacemaker circuitry.
- ◆ Specially designed lead for left ventricle introduced through coronary sinus and placed in a cardiac vein on surface of left ventricle.
- ◆ Challenging (or impossible) implant:
  - Variable venous anatomy.
  - Requires contrast medium to visualize cardiac veins.
  - Implant time longer than for typical pacemaker.
- ◆ Therapy delivered every heartbeat (100% ventricular pacing):
  - Coordinates ventricular contractions.
  - Improves hemodynamic status.
  - Results in paced QRS that may be narrower or different morphology compared to pacing right ventricle alone.

Temporary pacemaker

- ◆ A pacemaker may be used temporarily depending on the patient's condition.
- ◆ Temporary pacemakers commonly are used in emergencies to support the patient until the condition resolves:
  - Life-threatening bradyarrhythmias.
  - Evidence of decreased cardiac output (hypotension or syncope) after cardiac surgery.
  - High-grade heart block.
  - Need to overdrive atrial and ventricular tachyarrhythmias after cardiac surgery.
- ◆ A temporary pacemaker may serve as a bridge until a permanent pacemaker is inserted or replaced.
- ◆ These pacemakers may be invasive or noninvasive, but they don't require implantation.
- ◆ Look for an external pulse generator about the size of a small radio or telemetry box:
  - Powered by alkaline batteries.
  - Programmed by a touch pad or dials that control rate, output (milliamperes or mA), sensitivity, and AV interval.

Temporary pulse generator

The settings on a temporary pulse generator may be changed in a number of ways to meet the patient's specific needs. The illustration below shows a single-chamber temporary pulse generator and brief descriptions of its various parts.

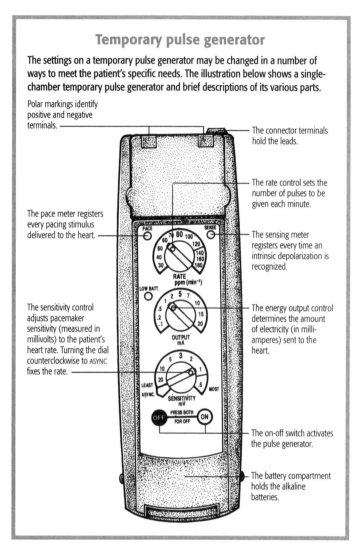

Polar markings identify positive and negative terminals.

The connector terminals hold the leads.

The rate control sets the number of pulses to be given each minute.

The pace meter registers every pacing stimulus delivered to the heart.

The sensing meter registers every time an intrinsic depolarization is recognized.

The sensitivity control adjusts pacemaker sensitivity (measured in millivolts) to the patient's heart rate. Turning the dial counterclockwise to ASYNC fixes the rate.

The energy output control determines the amount of electricity (in milli-amperes) sent to the heart.

The on-off switch activates the pulse generator.

The battery compartment holds the alkaline batteries.

– Positive and negative poles, two sets for atrium and ventricle for dual-chamber models and one set for single-chamber pacing.

◆ Several types are available: transvenous, epicardial, transcuta-neous, and transthoracic.

TRANSVENOUS PACING

◆ Usually easily tolerated by the patient.
◆ Most common and reliable type of temporary pacemaker.
◆ Can be inserted at the bedside or in a fluoroscopy suite.
◆ Characteristics of leadwires:
    – Balloon-tipped or stiff.
    – Inserted through a vein (subclavian, internal jugular, or femoral).
    – Advanced through a catheter into the right atrium or ventricle.
    – Connected to the pulse generator.
◆ Interventions after the pacing catheter is in place:
    – Threshold measurements.
    – Capture assessment.
    – Settings for rate, output, sensitivity, and mode.
    – Paced ECG for documentation of pacing rhythm.
    – Chest X-ray to rule out pneumothorax and determine lead position.
    – Bed rest with limited progression of activity depending on pacing catheter insertion site.

EPICARDIAL PACING

◆ Used for patients undergoing cardiac surgery.
◆ Characteristics of leadwires:
    – Tips attached to heart surface.
    – Brought through chest wall below the incision.
    – Attached to the pulse generator.
    – Removed several days after surgery or when the patient no longer needs them.

TRANSCUTANEOUS PACING

◆ Also known as external pacing.
◆ Quick and effective way to pace heart rhythm.
◆ Has become widely used in the past several years.
◆ Provides noninvasive VVI pacing.
◆ Uses external generator.
◆ Sends pacing impulses through the skin to the heart muscle.
◆ Allows adjustment of rate and output (mA).

◆ Position of electrode pads:
  – One on the patient's anterior chest wall to the right of the upper sternum but below the clavicle.
  – One on the back (anterior-posterior electrodes).
  – Possibly one to the left of the left nipple with the center of the electrode in the midaxillary line (also called the anterior-apex position).
◆ Commonly used in emergencies until transvenous pacemaker can be inserted.
◆ Physician not required for application.
◆ Variable patient tolerance:
  – Keep sedatives and analgesia readily available.
  – Watch for skin irritation.

TRANSTHORACIC PACING

◆ Provides temporary ventricular pacing.
◆ Used as a last resort during cardiac emergencies for patients with asystole or bradycardic arrest.
◆ Used rarely because of improvements in other temporary pacing methods.
◆ Requires insertion of a long needle into the right ventricle using subxiphoid approach.
◆ Pacing wire is guided into the endocardium through the needle, and positive and negative terminals are attached to the pacemaker generator.

Managing pacemaker therapy

Permanent pacemakers

◆ Use a systematic approach to assess pacemaker function for problems:
  – What's the mode?
  – What's the base rate and upper rate limit (maximum tracking or sensor rate)?
  – Are such features as mode switching or rate response activated?
  – Is the device a biventricular pacemaker?
  – Is the patient pacemaker-dependent?
  – Does the patient have signs and symptoms?

◆ Evaluate all sources of information:
  – Patient identification card issued by the pacemaker manufacturer.
  – Patient history.
  – Patient or family knowledge of device function.
  – Physician notes, printouts from programmer if available.
  – ECG observation.

◆ Review the patient's 12-lead ECG to evaluate pacemaker function. If unavailable, examine lead V_1 or MCL_1 instead.

◆ Select a monitoring lead that clearly shows the pacemaker spikes and compare at least two leads to verify what you observe.

◆ Remember: Visibility of spikes depends on pacing polarity and type of lead.

◆ Measure the rate and interpret the paced rhythm.

◆ Compare the morphology of paced and intrinsic complexes (traditional right ventricular pacing should produce a morphology similar to left bundle-branch block pattern).

◆ Differentiate between ventricular ectopy and paced activity.

◆ Look for information that tells you which chamber is paced and information about the pacemaker's sensing function.

◆ Monitor the patient's vital signs.

Distinguishing intermittent ventricular pacing from PVCs

Knowing whether your patient has an artificial pacemaker will help you avoid mistaking a ventricular paced beat for a premature venticular contraction (PVC). If your facility uses a monitoring system that eliminates artifact, make sure the monitor is set up correctly for a patient with a pacemaker. Otherwise, the pacemaker spikes may be eliminated as well.

If your patient has intermittent ventricular pacing, the paced ventricular complex will have a pacemaker spike preceding it, as shown in the shaded area of the top electrocardiogram

(ECG) strip. You may need to look in different leads for a bipolar pacemaker spike because it's small and may be difficult to see. What's more, the paced ventricular complex of a properly functioning pacemaker won't occur early or prematurely; it will occur only when the patient's own ventricular rate falls below the rate set for the pacemaker.

If your patient is having PVCs, they'll occur prematurely and won't have pacemaker spikes preceding them. Examples are shown in the shaded areas of the bottom ECG strip.

Intermittent ventricular pacing

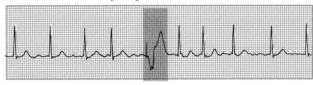

PVCs

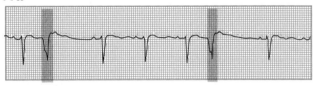

◆ Look for evidence of problems:
  – Decreased cardiac output (hypotension, chest pain, dyspnea, syncope).
  – Infection.
  – Pneumothorax.

– Abnormal electrical stimulation occurring in synchrony with the pacemaker.
– Pectoral muscle twitching.
– Hiccups (stimulation of diaphragm).
– Cardiac tamponade.

◆ Placing a magnet over the pulse generator makes the pacemaker temporarily revert to an asynchronous mode (safety mode) at a preset rate.

Assessing pacemaker function

When you apply a magnet to a pacemaker, the device reverts to a predefined (asynchronous) response mode that allows you to assess various aspects of pacemaker function. Specifically, you can accomplish the following:

◆ Determine which chambers are being paced.

◆ Assess capture.

◆ Provide emergency pacing if the device malfunctions.

◆ Ensure pacing despite electromagnetic interference.

◆ Assess battery life by checking the magnet rate – a predetermined rate that indicates the need for battery replacement.

Keep in mind, however, that you must know which implanted device the patient has before you consider using a magnet on it. The patient might have an implantable cardioverter-defibrillator (ICD), which only rarely is an appropriate target for magnet application.

It used to be relatively easy to tell a pacemaker from an ICD because of the difference in generator size and implant location. Today it isn't so easy. The generators are similar in size, and both kinds of devices are implanted under the skin of the patient's chest. What's more, a single device may perform multiple functions.

In general, you shouldn't apply a magnet to an ICD or a pacemaker-ICD combination. Applying a magnet to an ICD can cause an unexpected response because various responses can be programmed in or determined by the manufacturer. When directed, applying a magnet to an ICD usually suspends therapies for ventricular tachycardia and fibrillation while leaving bradycardia pacing active, which may be helpful in patients who receive multiple, inappropriate shocks. Some models may beep when exposed to a magnetic field.

PATIENT TEACHING

◆ Provide information to the patient about the following:
  – Function of pacemaker.
  – Related anatomy and physiology.
  – Patient's indication for pacemaker.
  – Postoperative care and routines.
◆ Provide discharge instructions, which usually include these topics:
  – Incision care.
  – Signs of pocket complications (hematoma, infection, bleeding).
  – Avoidance of heavy lifting or vigorous activity for 2 to 4 weeks.
  – Limited arm movement on side of pacemaker.
  – Medical follow-up.
  – Transtelephonic monitoring follow-up if indicated.
  – Identification card to be carried.
  – Procedure for taking pulse.
◆ Explain symptoms to report to physician:
  – Light-headedness, syncope, fatigue, palpitations, muscle stimulation, hiccups.
  – Slow (below the base rate) or unusually fast heart rate.
◆ Because today's pacemakers are well shielded from environmental interactions, explain that the patient can safely use the following:
  – Most common household appliances, including microwaves.
  – Cellular phones (on the side opposite the device).
  – Spark-ignited combustion engines (such as a leaf blower, lawnmower, automobile).
  – Office equipment (such as a computer, copier, fax machine).
  – Light shop equipment.
◆ Caution the patient to avoid close or prolonged exposure to potential sources of electromagnetic interference.

◆ Remind patient about travel-related issues:
– Metal detectors don't disturb device function but may detect the device.
– Handheld scanning tools shouldn't be used over the device or near it.
– An identification card may be needed to show security personnel.

Understanding electromagnetic interference

Electromagnetic interference (EMI) can wreak havoc on patients who have pacemakers or implanted cardioverter-defibrillators (ICDs). For someone with a pacemaker, EMI may inhibit pacing, cause asynchronous or unnecessary pacing, or mimic intrinsic cardiac activity. For someone with an ICD, EMI may mimic ventricular fibrillation, or it may prevent detection of a problem that needs treatment.

If your patient has a pacemaker or an ICD, review common sources of EMI and urge the patient to avoid them. These may include the following:
◆ Strong electromagnetic fields.
◆ Large generators and transformers.
◆ Arc and resistance welders.
◆ Large magnets.
◆ Motorized radiofrequency equipment.

EMI may present a risk in medical or hospital settings as well. Make sure your patient knows to notify all health care providers about the implanted device so the provider can evaluate the risk of therapies such as these:
◆ Magnetic resonance imaging (usually contraindicated).
◆ Radiation therapy (excluding diagnostic X-rays, such as mammograms, which typically are safe).
◆ Diathermy.
◆ Electrocautery.
◆ Transcutaneous electrical nerve stimulation therapy.

Temporary pacemakers

◆ Check stimulation and sensing thresholds daily because they increase over time.
◆ Assess the patient and pacemaker regularly to check for possible problems:
  – Failure to capture.
  – Undersensing.
  – Oversensing.
◆ Turn or reposition the patient carefully to prevent dislodgment of the leadwire.
◆ Follow recommended electrical safety precautions.
◆ Avoid microshocks to the patient by making sure that the bed and all electrical equipment is grounded properly and that all pacing wires and connections to temporary wires are insulated with moisture-proof material (such as a disposable glove).
◆ If there's no output (pacing is required but the pacemaker fails to stimulate the heart), take the following steps:
  – Verify that the pacemaker is on.
  – Check the output settings.
  – Change the pulse generator battery.
  – Change the pulse generator.
  – Check for disconnection or dislodgment of the pacing wire.
◆ Obtain a chest X-ray and assist the physician with repositioning the leadwire if required.

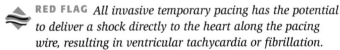 RED FLAG *All invasive temporary pacing has the potential to deliver a shock directly to the heart along the pacing wire, resulting in ventricular tachycardia or fibrillation.*

◆ Defibrillation and cardioversion (up to 400 joules) don't usually require that the pulse generator be disconnected.

◆ Look for evidence of problems:
  – Decreased cardiac output (hypotension, chest pain, dyspnea, syncope).
  – Infection.
  – Pneumothorax.
  – Abnormal electrical stimulation occurring in synchrony with the pacemaker.
  – Pectoral muscle twitching.
  – Hiccups (stimulation of diaphragm).
  – Cardiac tamponade.

PATIENT TEACHING

◆ Provide information to the patient about the following:
  – Function of pacemaker.
  – Related anatomy and physiology.
  – Patient's indication for pacemaker and potential need for permanent pacemaker.
  – Postprocedure care and pain management.
◆ Advise the patient not to get out of bed without assistance.
◆ Instruct him not to manipulate the pacemaker wires or pulse generator.
◆ Explain symptoms to report to the nurse:
  – Light-headedness, syncope, palpitations, muscle stimulation, or hiccups.
◆ Advise him to limit arm movement on the side of the pacemaker.

Pacemaker problems

◆ A malfunctioning pacemaker can lead to arrhythmias, syncope, hypotension, and decreased cardiac output.
◆ Pacemaker problems have some common causes:
  – Changes in the cardiac signal from MI or cardiomyopathy.
  – Disconnection or dislodgment of a lead.
  – Lead insulation failure.
  – Increased sensing threshold from edema or fibrosis at the electrode tip.
  – Pulse generator failure (sensing circuits).
  – Reversion of pacemaker to asynchronous pacing (safety mode).
◆ Certain pacemaker problems can lead to low cardiac output and loss of AV synchrony:
  – Failure to capture.
  – Failure to pace.
  – Undersensing.
  – Oversensing.

Failure to capture

◆ ECG shows a pacemaker spike without the appropriate atrial or ventricular response (spike without a complex), as shown below.

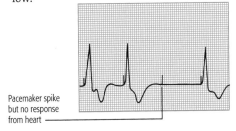

Pacemaker spike
but no response
from heart

◆ Patient may be asymptomatic or have signs of decreased cardiac output.
◆ Pacemaker is unable to stimulate the chamber.

◆ Problem may be caused by increased pacing thresholds related to certain situations:
- Metabolic or electrolyte imbalance.
- Antiarrhythmics.
- Fibrosis or edema at electrode tip.
◆ Problem may be caused by lead malfunction:
- Dislodged lead.
- Fractured or damaged lead.
- Perforation of myocardium by lead.
- Loose connection between lead and pulse generator.
◆ Related interventions may solve the problem:
- Treat metabolic disturbance.
- Replace damaged lead.
- Change pulse generator battery.
- Slowly increase output setting until capture occurs.

Failure to pace

◆ ECG shows no pacemaker activity when pacemaker activity should be evident, as shown below.

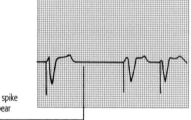

Pacemaker spike
should appear
here

◆ Magnet application yields no response. (It should cause asynchronous pacing.)
◆ Problem has several common causes:
- Depleted battery.
- Circuit failure.
- Lead malfunction.
- Inappropriate programming of sensing function.
- Electromagnetic interference.
◆ Failure to pace can lead to asystole or a severe decrease in cardiac output in pacemaker-dependent patients.

RED FLAG *If you think a pacemaker is failing to pace, a temporary pacemaker (transcutaneous or transvenous) should be used to prevent asystole.*

◆ Related interventions may solve the problem:
 – Replace pulse generator battery.
 – Replace pulse generator unit.
 – Adjust sensitivity setting.
 – Remove source of electromagnetic interference.

Undersensing

◆ ECG may show pacing spikes anywhere in the cycle, as shown below.

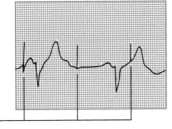

The pacemaker
fires anywhere in
the cycle

◆ A pacemaker spike may appear where intrinsic cardiac activity is already present.
◆ Patient may report feeling palpitations or skipped beats.
◆ Spikes are especially dangerous if they fall on the T wave because ventricular tachycardia or fibrillation may result.
◆ Problem has several common causes:
 – Battery failure.
 – Fracture of pacing leadwire.
 – Displacement of electrode tip.
 – "Cross-talk" between atrial and ventricular channels.
 – Electromagnetic interference mistaken for intrinsic signals.
◆ Related interventions may solve the problem:
 – Replace the pulse generator battery.
 – Replace the leadwires.
 – Adjust the sensitivity setting.

Oversensing

♦ If the pacemaker is too sensitive, it can misinterpret muscle movement or extracardiac events as intrinsic cardiac electrical activity and pacing won't occur when it's needed.

♦ In DDD mode, fast rates may occur if the ventricle tracks extracardiac events as P waves.

♦ Pacing doesn't occur when the intrinsic rate drops below the lower set rate or pacing may not be observed in one or both chambers.

♦ AV synchrony can be lost.

♦ Problem has several common causes:
  – T-wave sensing.
  – Electromagnetic interference.
  – Lead malfunction.

♦ Related interventions may solve the problem:
  – Adjust the sensitivity setting.
  – Avoid electromagnetic interference.
  – Replace the leadwire.

Implantable cardioverter-defibrillators

- Implanted electronic device used mainly for life-threatening arrhythmias.
- Programmed to automatically detect many different arrhythmias:
  - Ventricular tachycardia.
  - Ventricular fibrillation.
  - Bradycardia.
- Automatically responds with appropriate therapy.
- Widening indications over the past decade.
- Originally implanted as secondary prevention after patient survived certain arrhythmias:
  - Sudden death from ventricular fibrillation.
  - Hemodynamically unstable ventricular tachycardia.
- Now used as primary prevention in patients at high risk for ventricular arrhythmias:
  - Coronary disease and low ejection fraction.
  - Hypertrophic cardiomyopathy.
  - Dilated cardiomyopathy with low ejection fraction.
- Detection rate:
  - Defines what the device recognizes as ventricular tachycardia or fibrillation.
  - Primary detection criterion.
  - May have separate detection rates (zones) for ventricular tachycardia and fibrillation.
  - Requires a rate sustained for a predetermined number of cycles.
- Can deliver multitiered therapies:
  - Defibrillation (always programmed).
  - Cardioversion (may be used for ventricular tachycardia).
  - Antitachycardia pacing (may be used for ventricular tachycardia).
  - Postshock pacing support (always programmed).
  - Cardiac resynchronization therapy (also known as biventricular pacing)
  - Bradycardia pacing.

Implantable cardioverter-defibrillator review

An implantable cardioverter-defibrillator (ICD) has a programmable pulse generator and lead system that monitors the heart's activity, detects ventricular arrhythmias and other tachyarrhythmias, and responds with appropriate therapies. The range of therapies includes antitachycardia and antibradycardia pacing, cardioversion, and defibrillation. Newer defibrillators can also pace both atrium and ventricle.

Implantation of an ICD is similar to that of a permanent pacemaker. The cardiologist positions the lead (or leads) transvenously in the endocardium of the right ventricle (and the right atrium, if both chambers need pacing). The lead connects to a generator box implanted in the right or left upper chest near the clavicle.

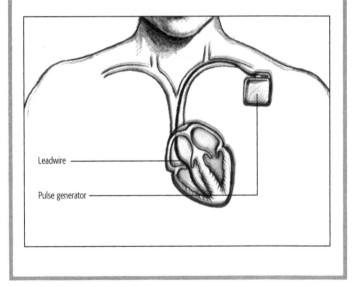

Leadwire

Pulse generator

Types of ICD therapies

An implantable cardioverter-defibrillator (ICD) can deliver a range of therapies depending on how the device is programmed and the arrhythmia it detects. Therapies include antitachycardia pacing, cardioversion, defibrillation, and bradycardia pacing.

Therapy	Description
Antitachycardia pacing	A series of small, rapid electrical pacing pulses used to interrupt ventricular tachycardia (VT) and return the heart to its normal rhythm. Antitachycardia pacing isn't appropriate for all patients and begins only after appropriate electrophysiology studies.
Cardioversion	A low- or high-energy shock (up to 35 joules) timed to the R wave to terminate VT and return the heart to its normal rhythm.
Defibrillation	A high-energy shock (up to 35 joules) to the heart to terminate ventricular fibrillation and return the heart to its normal rhythm.
Bradycardia pacing	Electrical pacing pulses used when natural electrical signals are too slow. Most ICDs pace one chamber (VVI pacing) of the heart at a preset rate. Some can sense and pace both chambers (DDD pacing).

Managing an ICD

◆ Know the device and how it's programmed:
  – Type and model of ICD.
  – Status of the device (on or off).
  – Detection rates.
  – Types of therapies that will be delivered and when.
◆ Evaluate the appropriateness of ICD shocks:
  – Number of isolated and multiple shocks.
  – Situation and activity related to shocks.
  – Patient symptoms.
  – ECG rhythm.
  – Drugs taken.
◆ Keep in mind that shocks may not occur despite ventricular tachycardia or fibrillation under certain circumstances:
  – If the heart rate is less than the detection rate.
  – If there's a lead or circuitry problem.
  – If therapy is suspended or turned off.
  – If the battery is depleted.

 RED FLAG *If cardiac arrest occurs in a patient with an ICD, cardiopulmonary resuscitation (CPR) and advanced cardiac life support should be used immediately.*

◆ If the patient needs external defibrillation, take the following steps:
  – Position the paddles as far from the device as possible.
  – Alternatively, use anterior-posterior position.
  – Anticipate that defibrillation will result in "power on reset" and reversion to nominal settings.
  – Programming of device should be verified with the programmer.
◆ Keep in mind that shocks can occur without ventricular tachycardia or fibrillation under certain circumstances:
  – When the rate in sinus tachycardia ventures into the ventricular tachycardia zone.
  – When noise is detected on the sensing lead (from electromagnetic interference or lead dysfunction).
  – When the patient develops atrial fibrillation.

◆ Keep in mind that multiple shocks may occur in certain circumstances:

 – When the patient has persistent or recurrent ventricular tachycardia or fibrillation.

 – When the device malfunctions.

◆ Multiple shocks indicate a medical emergency, and the patient may require adjunct treatment:

 – CPR.

 – External defibrillation.

 – Drugs such as lidocaine, amiodarone, procainamide.

 – Suspension of tachyarrhythmia therapy by magnet application or reprogramming of device.

◆ Look for evidence of problems:

 – Decreased cardiac output (hypotension, chest pain, dyspnea, syncope).

 – Infection.

 – Pneumothorax.

 – Abnormal electrical stimulation occurring in synchrony with the pacemaker.

 – Pectoral muscle twitching.

 – Hiccups (stimulation of diaphragm).

 – Cardiac tamponade.

PATIENT TEACHING

◆ Provide teaching similar to that for patients with pacemakers, plus additional teaching for special needs.
  – Patient may have experienced cardiac arrest.
  – Patient may still be at risk for syncope.
  – Diagnosis may be associated with multiple life-changing components.
◆ Risk of syncope may continue because the device treats arrhythmia but doesn't prevent ventricular tachycardia or fibrillation from occurring.
◆ Explain driving restrictions, if ordered.
◆ Tell the patient and family what to do if the device delivers a shock.
◆ Tell the patient what to do if symptoms of arrhythmia develop but the device doesn't deliver treatment:
  – Notify the physician.
  – Activate local emergency medical service, as appropriate.
  – Suggest training in CPR for family members.

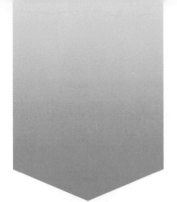

10

Basic 12-lead electrocardiography

◆ A 12-lead ECG is a diagnostic test that does the following:
  – Helps identify such pathologic conditions as angina and acute myocardial infarction.
  – Gives a more complete view of the heart's electrical activity than a rhythm strip.
  – Allows more effective assessment of left ventricular function than a rhythm strip.
◆ The test results are viewed with other patient data:
  – History.
  – Physical assessment findings.
  – Laboratory test results.
  – Diagnostic study results.
  – Drug regimen.

Understanding ECG leads and electrical axes

◆ Twelve leads provide 12 different views of the heart's electrical activity.
◆ Each lead transmits information about a different area of the heart.
◆ Waveforms obtained from each lead vary based on the location of the lead in relation to the wave of depolarization passing through the myocardium.
◆ The 12 leads include six limb leads and six precordial leads.

Limb leads

◆ Record electrical activity in the heart's frontal plane:
  – A view through the middle of the heart from top to bottom.
◆ Record electrical activity from the anterior to the posterior axes.
◆ Include three bipolar limb leads (I, II, III).
◆ Include three unipolar augmented limb leads (aV_R, aV_L, and aV_F).

ECG leads

Each of the leads on a 12-lead electrocardiograph (ECG) views the heart from a different angle. These illustrations show the direction of electrical activity (depolarization) monitored by each lead and the 12 views of the heart.

Views reflected on a 12-lead ECG	Lead	View of the heart
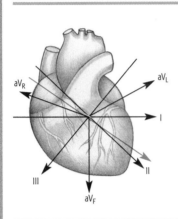	*Standard limb leads (bipolar)*	
	I	Lateral wall
	II	Inferior wall
	III	Inferior wall
	Augmented limb leads (unipolar)	
	aV_R	No specific view
	aV_L	Lateral wall
	aV_F	Inferior wall
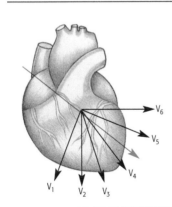	*Precordial, or chest, leads (unipolar)*	
	V_1	Septal wall
	V_2	Septal wall
	V_3	Anterior wall
	V_4	Anterior wall
	V_5	Lateral wall
	V_6	Lateral wall

Precordial leads

◆ Also known as chest leads.
◆ Provide information on electrical activity in the heart's horizontal plane:
  – A transverse view through the middle of the heart, dividing it into upper and lower portions.
◆ Record electrical activity from either a superior or an inferior approach
◆ Standard precordial leads:
  – Six unipolar leads.
  – V_1, V_2, V_3, V_4, V_5, and V_6.
  – Allow evaluation of left ventricle.
◆ Right precordial leads:
  – Six unipolar leads.
  – V_1R, V_2R, V_3R, V_4R, V_5R, and V_6R.
  – Allow evaluation of right ventricle.

Posterior leads

◆ Lung and muscle barriers prevent usual chest leads from seeing and recording damage on posterior surface of heart.
◆ Posterior leads:
  – Three unipolar leads.
  – V_7, V_8, and V_9.
  – Allow assessment of posterior heart surface.

Electrical axes

◆ Recorded by a 12-lead electrocardiograph (ECG).
◆ Refer to the force and direction of the wave of depolarization through the heart.
◆ May be called the mean instantaneous vector, which refers to mean of small electrical forces (instantaneous vectors) generated by impulses traveling through heart.
◆ May be called the mean QRS vector.
◆ Impulses in a healthy heart:
  – Originate in the sinoatrial node, travel through the atria to the atrioventricular node, and travel to the ventricles.
  – Move downward and to the left, the direction of a normal axis.
◆ Impulses in an unhealthy heart:
  – Variable axis direction.
  – Movement of electrical activity away from areas of damage or necrosis and toward areas of hypertrophy.

Preparing for a 12-lead ECG

◆ Gather all needed supplies.
◆ Explain the procedure to the patient.
◆ Answer the patient's questions.
◆ Ask the patient to lie supine in the center of the bed with arms at sides.
◆ If the patient can't tolerate lying flat, raise the head of the bed to semi-Fowler's position.
◆ Ensure privacy.
◆ Expose the patient's arms, legs, and chest.
◆ Drape the patient for comfort.

Selecting lead sites

◆ Choose areas that are flat and fleshy, not muscular or bony.
◆ As needed, takes steps to enhance electrode contact with the skin:
  – Clip excessively hairy areas.
  – Remove excess oil and other substances from the skin.
◆ To ensure an accurate recording, the electrodes must be applied correctly.

 RED FLAG *Inaccurate placement of an electrode by more than ³⁄₅″ (1.5 cm) from its correct position may lead to inaccurate waveforms and an incorrect ECG interpretation.*

Placing leads

LIMB LEADS

◆ Place electrodes on both of the patient's arms and on the left leg.
◆ Place an electrode on the right leg. (This is a ground that doesn't contribute to the waveform.)

Limb lead placement

Proper lead placement is critical for accurate recording of cardiac rhythms. These drawings show correct electrode placement for the six limb leads. RA stands for right arm; LA, left arm; RL, right leg; and LL, left leg. The plus sign (+) indicates the positive pole, the minus sign (–) indicates the negative pole, and G indicates the ground. Below each drawing is a sample ECG strip for that lead.

Lead I

Connects the right arm (negative pole) with the left arm (positive pole).

Lead II

Connects the right arm (negative pole) with the left leg (positive pole).

Lead III

Connects the left arm (negative pole) with the left leg (positive pole).

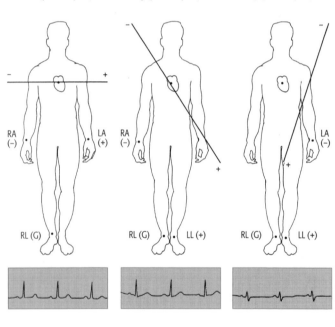

Lead aV_R

Connects the right arm (positive pole) with the heart (negative pole).

Lead aV_L

Connects the left arm (positive pole) with the heart (negative pole)

Lead aV_F

Connects the left leg (positive pole) with the heart (negative pole).

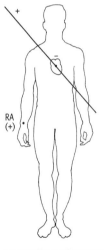

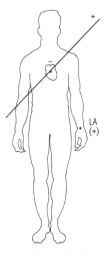

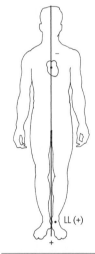

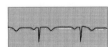

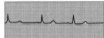

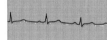

Precordial lead placement

To record a 12-lead electrocardiogram, place electrodes on the patient's arms and legs and a ground lead on the patient's right leg. The three standard limb leads (I, II, and III) and the three augmented leads (aV_R, aV_L, and aV_F) are recorded using these electrodes. Then, to record the precordial chest leads, place electrodes as follows:

- V_1 – fourth intercostal space (ICS), right sternal border
- V_2 – fourth ICS, left sternal border
- V_3 – midway between V_2 and V_4
- V_4 – fifth ICS, left midclavicular line
- V_5 – fifth ICS, left anterior axillary line
- V_6 – fifth ICS, left midaxillary line.

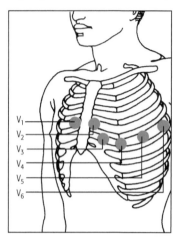

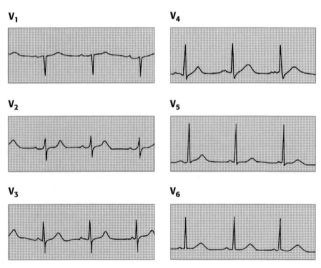

Right precordial lead placement

Right precordial leads can provide specific information about the function of the right ventricle. Place the six leads on the right side of the chest in a mirror image of the standard precordial lead placement, as shown here.

V_1R: fourth intercostal space (ICS), left sternal border
V_2R: fourth ICS, right sternal border
V_3R: halfway between V_2R and V_4R
V_4R: fifth ICS, right midclavicular line
V_5R: fifth ICS, right anterior axillary line
V_6R: fifth ICS, right midaxillary line

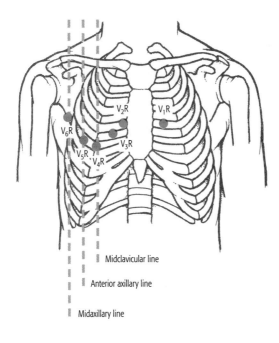

Midclavicular line

Anterior axillary line

Midaxillary line

Posterior lead placement

Posterior leads can be used to assess the posterior side of the heart. To ensure an accurate reading, make sure the posterior electrodes V_7, V_8, and V_9 are placed at the same horizontal level as the V_6 lead at the fifth intercostal space. Place lead V_7 at the posterior axillary line, lead V_9 at the paraspinal line, and lead V_8 halfway between leads V_7 and V_9.

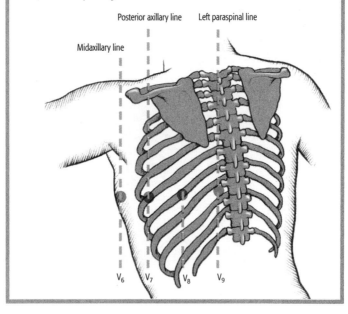

Recording the ECG

◆ Plug the cord of the ECG machine into a grounded outlet unless the machine operates on a charged battery and doesn't
need to be plugged in.

◆ Turn on the machine.

◆ Enter the patient's identification data, if necessary.

◆ Place all of the electrodes on the patient.

◆ Make sure all leads are securely attached.

◆ Instruct the patient to relax, lie still, breathe normally, and re-
frain from talking during the recording to prevent distortion of
the ECG tracing.

◆ Make sure that the ECG paper speed selector is set to the standard 25 mm per second.

◆ Start recording the ECG by pressing the appropriate button on
the machine.

◆ Observe the quality of the tracing.

◆ Turn off the machine when it finishes the recording.

◆ Remove the electrodes and clean the patient's skin.

Reading the ECG

♦ Make sure the printout shows pertinent information:
  – Patient's name.
  – Patient's room number.
  – Patient's medical record number, if appropriate.
  – Date.
  – Time.
  – Physician's name.
  – Patient's heart rate.
  – Wave durations (measured in seconds).
  – Lead that's being recorded.
♦ Make sure special circumstances are noted, as needed:
  – Episodes of chest pain.
  – Abnormal electrolyte levels.
  – Related drug treatment.
  – Abnormal placement of electrodes.
  – Presence of an artificial pacemaker.
  – Whether a magnet was used while the ECG was obtained.
♦ Keep in mind important facts about ECG recordings.
  – They're legal documents.
  – They belong in the patient's medical record.
  – They must be saved for future reference and comparison with baseline strips.

Understanding a multichannel ECG recording

The top of a 12-lead electrocardiogram (ECG) recording typically includes patient identification information and an interpretation by the machine. A rhythm strip commonly appears at the bottom of the recording.

On the recording, look for standardization marks, normally 10 small squares in height. If the patient has high-voltage complexes, the marks will be half as high. You'll also notice that lead markers separate the lead recordings on the paper and that each lead is named.

Familiarize yourself with the way the leads are laid out on the recording so you can interpret the ECG results more quickly and accurately.

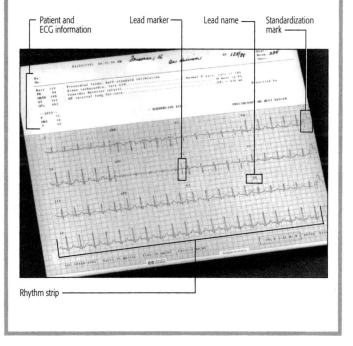

Patient and ECG information   Lead marker   Lead name   Standardization mark

Rhythm strip

Transtelephonic cardiac monitoring

Patients with transient cardiac symptoms such as palpitations, dizziness, syncope, confusion, paroxysmal dyspnea, and atypical chest pain once faced an uphill battle for a diagnosis. Because transient symptoms rarely arise during scheduled health care visits, patients commonly had to be admitted and monitored until the symptoms surfaced.

Now, with the advent of transtelephonic monitoring (TTM), patients can send electrocardiogram (ECG) information by phone to a monitoring center whenever the symptoms hit. Because patients can keep the equipment for long periods of time, even rare symptoms can be recorded and evaluated. TTM is especially valuable for assessing the effects of drugs and for diagnosing and managing paroxysmal arrhythmias, thus eliminating the need for potentially lengthy hospital stays.

TTM process

TTM requires three main pieces of equipment:
- An ECG recorder-transmitter.
- A standard telephone line.
- A receiver.

The recorder-transmitter converts cardiac electrical activity to acoustic waves and sends them through a telephone line to a receiver, which converts the waves and records them on ECG paper.

Recorder-transmitters come in several models and are still evolving. One model uses two electrodes applied to the finger and chest to produce a tracing similar to that of a standard 12-lead ECG. Another model is about the size of a credit card. When symptoms start, the patient holds the card firmly to the center of his chest and pushes the start button. Four electrodes on the back of the card sense electrical activity and record and store up to 30 seconds of activity.

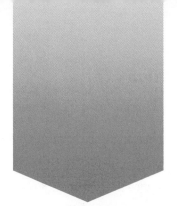

11

Advanced electrocardiography

Steps in ECG interpretation

◆ Check the electrocardiogram (ECG) tracing to see if it's technically correct.
◆ Use a systematic approach for interpretation, and compare with the patient's previous ECG.
◆ Quickly scan limb leads I, II, and III.
  – R-wave voltage in lead II should equal the sum of the R-wave voltage in leads I and III.
  – Lead aV_R is typically negative.
◆ Locate the lead markers.
◆ Check the standardization markings (1 millivolt or 10 mm).
◆ Assess the patient's heart rate and rhythm.
◆ Determine the heart's electrical axis.
  – The average direction of the heart's electrical activity during ventricular depolarization.
  – Determined by examining waveforms recorded from the six frontal plane leads: I, II, III, aV_R, aV_L, and aV_F.
  – May use quadrant method or degree method.
◆ Examine limb leads I, II, and III.
  – R wave: Taller in lead II than in lead I; in lead III, a smaller version of R wave in lead I.
  – P wave or QRS complex: May be inverted.
  – ST segment: Flat.

R-wave progression

R waves should progress normally through the precordial leads. Note that the R wave in this strip is the first positive deflection in the QRS complex. Also note that the S wave gets smaller, or regresses, from lead V_1 to V_6 until it finally disappears.

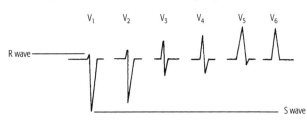

- T wave: Upright.
- Pathologic Q waves: Absent.

◆ Examine limb leads aV_L, aV_F, and aV_R.
- Leads aV_L and aV_F: Possibly similar tracings but lead aV_F should have taller P and R waves.
- P wave, QRS complex, and T wave: Deflect downward in lead aV_R.

◆ Examine the R wave in the precordial leads.
- Progressively taller from lead V_1 to V_5.
- Slightly smaller in lead V_6.

◆ Examine the S wave in the precordial leads.
- Extremely deep in lead V_1.
- Progressively more shallow.
- Usually gone by lead V_5.

Waveform abnormalities

◆ The location of changes in each lead can determine the area of the heart affected.

P WAVES

◆ Peaked, notched, or enlarged P waves may signify atrial hypertrophy or enlargement.
◆ Inverted P waves may signify retrograde conduction.
◆ Varying P waves signify an impulse originating from different sites, as with irritable atrial tissue.
◆ Absent P waves may signify conduction by a route other than the sinoatrial (SA) node.

PR INTERVALS

◆ Short PR intervals (less than 0.12 second) signify impulses originating somewhere other than the SA node, as in junctional arrhythmias or preexcitation syndromes.
◆ Prolonged PR intervals (greater than 0.20 seconds) signify a conduction delay, as in heart block or digoxin toxicity.

QRS COMPLEX

◆ A duration greater than 0.12 second may signify ventricular conduction.
◆ One or more missing QRS complexes may signify atrioventricular (AV) block or ventricular standstill.

Q WAVE

◆ A Q wave is considered abnormal if it has a depth greater than 4 mm or a height of one-fourth of the R wave.
◆ Abnormal Q waves signify myocardial necrosis.
◆ Abnormal Q waves develop when damaged tissue prevents depolarization from following its normal path.

ST SEGMENT

◆ The ST segment is considered abnormal if it's elevated more than 1 mm above the baseline, depressed more than 0.5 mm below the baseline, or both.

◆ It will be elevated in leads facing an injured area.
◆ It will be depressed in leads facing away from the injured area.

T WAVE

◆ Tall, peaked, or tented T waves may signify myocardial injury or hyperkalemia.
◆ Inverted T waves may signify myocardial ischemia.

QT INTERVAL

◆ A prolonged QT interval (greater than 0.44 second) indicates prolonged ventricular repolarization and congenital prolonged QT syndrome.
◆ A short QT interval (less than 0.36 second) may result from digoxin toxicity or hypercalcemia.

Electrical axis deviation

◆ Finding the patient's electrical axis can help confirm a diagnosis.

◆ Axis deviation occurs when electrical activity in the heart moves away from areas of damage or necrosis.

◆ Normal: Between 0 and 90 degrees. (Some sources consider –30 to 90 degrees to be normal.)

◆ Right axis deviation: Between 90 and 180 degrees.

◆ Left axis deviation: Between 0 and –90 degrees. (Some sources consider –30 to –90 degrees to be left axis deviation.)

◆ Extreme axis deviation (indeterminate axis): Between –180 and –90 degrees.

Hexaxial reference system

The hexaxial reference system consists of six bisecting lines, each representing one of the six limb leads, and a circle representing the heart. The intersection of all lines divides the circle into equal, 30-degree segments.

Shifting degrees

Note that 0 degrees appears at the 3 o'clock position (positive pole lead I). Moving counterclockwise, the degrees become increasingly negative until reaching ±180 degrees at the 9 o'clock position (negative pole lead I).

The bottom half of the circle contains the corresponding positive degrees. However, a positive-degree designation doesn't necessarily mean that the pole is positive.

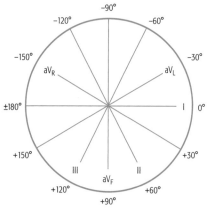

Electrial axis determination: Quadrant method

This chart will help you quickly determine the direction of a patient's electrical axis. Observe the deflections of the QRS complexes in leads I and aV_F. Lead I indicates whether impulses are moving to the right or left, and lead aV_F indicates whether they're moving up or down. Then check the chart to determine whether the patient's axis is normal or has a left, right, or extreme axis deviation.

◆ Normal axis: QRS-complex deflection is positive or upright in both leads.
◆ Left axis deviation: Lead I is upright and lead aV_F points down.
◆ Right axis deviation: Lead I points down and lead aV_F is upright.
◆ Extreme axis deviation: Both waves point down.

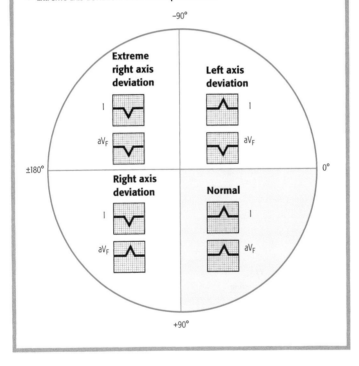

Electrical axis determination: Degree method

A more precise axis calculation, the degree method provides an exact measurement of the electrical axis. It allows you to identify a patient's electrical axis by degrees on the hexaxial system, not just by quadrant. It also allows you to determine the axis even if the QRS complex isn't clearly positive or negative in leads I and aV_F. To use this method, take the following steps.

Step 1

Identify the limb lead with the smallest QRS complex or the equiphasic QRS complex. In this example, it's lead III.

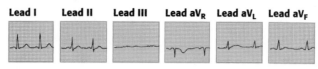

| Lead I | Lead II | Lead III | Lead aV_R | Lead aV_L | Lead aV_F |

Step 2

Locate the axis for lead III on the hexaxial diagram. Then find the axis perpendicular to it, which is the axis for lead aV_R.

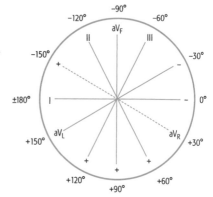

Step 3

Now, examine the QRS complex in lead aV_R, noting whether the deflection is positive or negative. As you can see, the QRS complex for this lead is negative, indicating that the current is moving toward the negative pole of aV_R, which is in the right lower quadrant at +30 degrees on the hexaxial diagram. So the electrical axis here is normal at +30 degrees.

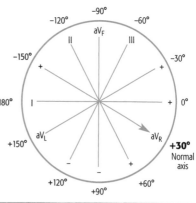

+30°
Normal axis

Causes of axis deviation

◆ Factors that influence axis location include the position of the heart in the chest, heart size, body size, and conduction pathways.

◆ Deviation isn't always cardiac in origin, and it isn't always an abnormality. For example, infants and children normally have right axis deviation and pregnant women normally have left axis deviation.

LEFT AXIS DEVIATION

◆ May be a normal variation.
◆ Causes:
  – Aging.
  – Aortic stenosis.
  – Inferior-wall myocardial infarction (MI).
  – Left anterior hemiblock.
  – Left bundle-branch block.
  – Left ventricular hypertrophy.
  – Mechanical shifts (ascites, pregnancy, tumors).
  – Wolff-Parkinson-White (WPW) syndrome.

RIGHT AXIS DEVIATION

◆ May be a normal variation.
◆ Causes:
  – Emphysema.
  – Lateral-wall MI.
  – Left posterior hemiblock.
  – Pulmonary hypertension.
  – Pulmonic stenosis.
  – Right bundle-branch block.
  – Right ventricular hypertrophy.

Disorders affecting the 12-lead ECG

♦ 12-lead ECG is used to assist in the diagnosis of certain conditions:
  – Angina, including Prinzmetal's variant angina.
  – MI.
  – Pericarditis.
  – Left ventricular hypertrophy.
  – Bundle-branch block.

Angina

♦ A symptom of myocardial ischemia.
♦ Occurs when the myocardium needs more oxygen than the coronary arteries can deliver.
♦ Stable angina:
  – Provoked by exertion or stress.
  – Usually lasts 2 to 10 minutes.
  – Typically relieved by rest.
  – Repeats in this pattern.
♦ Unstable angina:
  – Provoked more easily than stable angina.
  – Commonly wakes the patient.
  – Unpredictable.
  – Worsens over time.

ECG changes in angina

Illustrated below are some classic electrocardiogram (ECG) changes involving the T wave and ST segment that you may see when monitoring a patient with angina.

Peaked T wave	Flattened T wave	T-wave inversion	ST-segment depression with T-wave inversion	ST-segment depression without T-wave inversion

  – Classified as an acute coronary syndrome with MI.
  – Treated as a medical emergency.
  – Usually portends an MI.
◆ Prinzmetal's variant angina:
  – A relatively uncommon form of unstable angina.
  – Usually occurs at rest or wakes the patient from sleep.

ECG changes in Prinzmetal's angina

This illustration shows a 12-lead electrocardiogram (ECG) of a patient with Prinzmetal's angina. Marked ST-segment elevations appear in leads that are monitoring the heart area where the coronary artery spasm occurs. The elevation occurs during chest pain and resolves when pain subsides. T waves are usually of normal size and configuration.

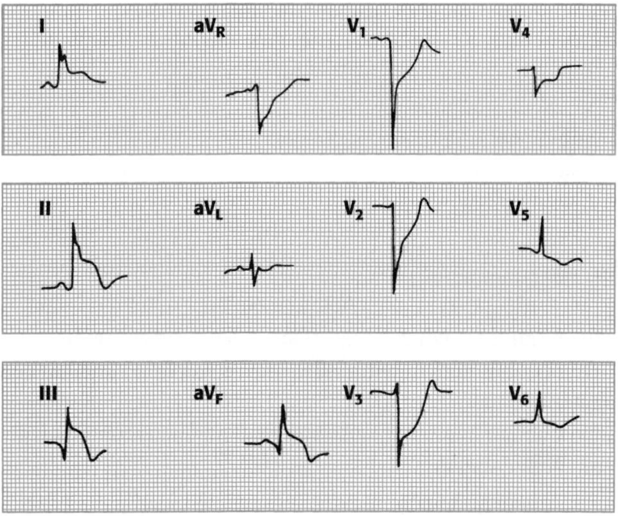

CAUSES

◆ Decreased blood flow results from narrowing of the arteries from coronary artery disease (CAD), which may be complicated by platelet clumping, thrombus formation, and vasospasm.
◆ In Prinzmetal's variant angina, vasospasm results from a focal episodic spasm of a coronary artery, with or without an obstructing coronary artery lesion.

SIGNS AND SYMPTOMS

◆ Stable angina:
   – Predictable pain pattern.
   – Substernal or precrodial burning, squeezing, or tightness.
   – May radiate to left arm, neck, or jaw.
   – Relieved by nitrates or rest.
◆ Unstable angina:
   – Chest pain that may or may not radiate.
   – Greater intensity and duration than stable angina.
   – Also pallor, diaphoresis, nausea, or anxiety.
◆ Prinzmetal's angina:
   – Substernal chest pain from heaviness to crushing discomfort.
   – Usually occurs at rest or wakes the patient from sleep.
   – Also dyspnea, nausea, vomiting, or diaphoresis.

 Interventions

◆ Give nitrates to reduce myocardial oxygen consumption.
◆ Give beta blockers to reduce the heart's workload and oxygen demands.
◆ Give calcium channel blockers to treat angina caused by coronary artery spasm.
◆ Give antiplatelet drugs to minimize platelet aggregation and the risk of coronary occlusion.
◆ Give antilipemic drugs to reduce elevated serum cholesterol or triglycerides levels.
◆ If the patient has continued unstable angina or acute chest pain or has had an invasive cardiac procedure, give glycoprotein IIb/IIIa inhibitors to reduce platelet aggregation.
◆ Anticipate coronary artery bypass surgery or percutaneous transluminal coronary angioplasty for obstructive lesions.

Myocardial infarction

◆ MI is categorized as an acute coronary syndrome.

◆ Reduced blood flow through one or more coronary arteries causes myocardial ischemia and necrosis.

◆ Damage usually occurs in the left ventricle, although the location varies with the coronary artery affected.

◆ As long as the myocardium is deprived of oxygen-rich blood, the ECG will reflect three pathologic changes: ischemia, injury, and infarction.

◆ In a non–Q-wave MI, abnormalities may include non–ST-segment elevation or ST-segment depression.

◆ In a Q-wave MI, abnormalities may include ST-segment elevation and Q waves, which represent scarring and necrosis.

Zones of MI

Myocardial infarction (MI) has a central area of necrosis surrounded by a zone of injury that may recover if revascularization occurs. This zone of injury is surrounded by an outer zone of reversible ischemia. Each zone produces characteristic electrocardiogram changes.

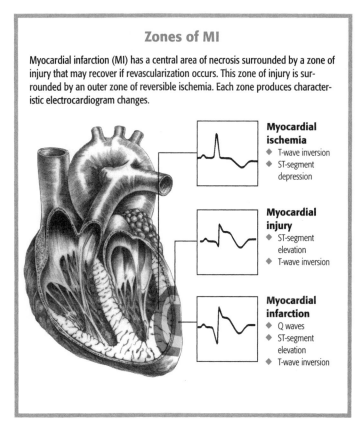

Myocardial ischemia
◆ T-wave inversion
◆ ST-segment depression

Myocardial injury
◆ ST-segment elevation
◆ T-wave inversion

Myocardial infarction
◆ Q waves
◆ ST-segment elevation
◆ T-wave inversion

Locating myocardial damage

After you've noted characteristic lead changes in an acute myocardial infarction, use this table to identify the areas of damage. Match the lead changes (ST elevation, abnormal Q waves) in the second column with the affected wall in the first column and the artery involved in the third column. The fourth column shows reciprocal lead changes.

Wall affected	Leads	Artery involved	Reciprocal changes
Anterior	V_2, V_3, V_4	Left coronary artery, left anterior descending (LAD)	II, III, aV_F
Anterolateral	I, aV_L, V_3, V_4, V_5, V_6	LAD and diagonal branches, circumflex and marginal branches	II, III, aV_F
Anteroseptal	V_1, V_2, V_3, V_4	LAD	None
Inferior	II, III, aV_F	Right coronary artery (RCA)	I, aV_L
Lateral	I, aV_L, V_5, V_6	Circumflex branch of left coronary artery	II, III, aV_F
Posterior	V_8, V_9	RCA or circumflex	V_1, V_2, V_3, V_4 (R greater than S in V_1 and V_2, ST-segment depression, elevated T wave)
Right ventricular	V_{4R}, V_{5R}, V_{6R}	RCA	None

CAUSES

◆ Atherosclerosis:
  – Formation of plaque, an unstable and lipid-rich substance.
  – Subsequent rupture or erosion of plaque, resulting in platelet adhesion, fibrin clot formation, and activation of thrombin.
◆ Embolus.
◆ Risk factors:
  – Diabetes.
  – Family history of heart disease.
  – High-fat, high-carbohydrate diet.
  – Hyperlipoproteinemia.
  – Hypertension.
  – Menopause.
  – Obesity.
  – Sedentary lifestyle.
  – Smoking.
  – Stress.

SIGNS AND SYMPTOMS

◆ Chest pain:
  – Severe, persistent, burning, squeezing, or crushing.
  – Usually substernal or precordial.
  – May radiate to left arm, neck, jaw, or shoulder blade.
  – Lasts at least 20 minutes and may persist for several hours.
  – Unrelieved by rest.
◆ Other signs and symptoms:
  – Anxiety.
  – Cool extremities.
  – Fatigue.
  – Feeling of impending doom.
  – Hypertension.
  – Hypotension.
  – Nausea.
  – Shortness of breath.
  – Vomiting.
◆ Atypical presentation:
  – More likely in women, elderly patients, and patients with diabetes.

– May include vague or absent chest discomfort; jaw, back or shoulder pain; shortness of breath; fatigue; or abdominal discomfort.

Interventions

RED FLAG *If a patient develops chest pain, take immediate measures to decrease cardiac workload and increase oxygen supply to the myocardium. These measures include rest, pain relief, and supplemental oxygen.*

◆ If symptoms started during previous 3 hours, prepare for thrombolytic therapy (unless contraindicated) to restore vessel patency and minimize necrosis.

◆ Give oxygen to increase oxygenation of blood.

◆ Give nitroglycerin sublingually to relieve chest pain (unless systolic blood pressure is less than 90 mm Hg or heart rate is less than 50 or more than 100 beats/minute).

◆ Give morphine to relieve pain.

◆ Give aspirin to inhibit platelet aggregation.

◆ If the patient received tissue plasminogen activator, give I.V. heparin to promote patency in the affected coronary artery.

◆ If the patient has an arrhythmia, prepare for use of antiarrhythmics, transcutaneous pacing patches (or transvenous pacemaker), defibrillation, or epinephrine.

◆ A patient without hypotension, bradycardia, or excessive tachycardia may receive I.V. nitroglycerin for 24 to 48 hours to reduce afterload and preload and relieve chest pain.

◆ If the patient has continued unstable angina or acute chest pain or has had an invasive cardiac procedure, give glycoprotein IIb/IIIa inhibitors to reduce platelet aggregation.

◆ Percutaneous transluminal angioplasty, stent placement, coronary artery atherectomy, or coronary artery bypass graft may be used to open blocked or narrowed arteries.

Recognizing an anterior-wall MI

This 12-lead electrocardiogram shows typical characteristics (V_2, V_3, V_4) of an anterior-wall myocardial infarction (MI). Note that the R waves don't progress through the precordial leads. Also note the ST-segment elevation in leads V_2 and V_3. As expected, the reciprocal leads II, III, and aV_F show slight ST-segment depression.

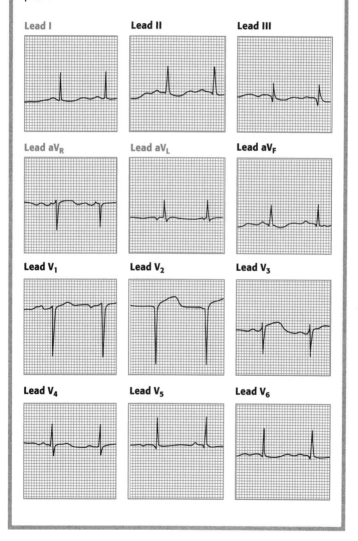

Recognizing an anteroseptal-wall MI

This 12-lead electrcardiogram shows typical characteristics of an anteroseptal-wall myocardial infarction (MI). Note the loss of R in leads V_1 and V_2. Also note the ST-segment elevation in leads V_1 to V_4.

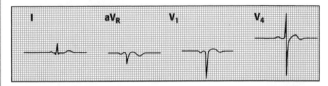

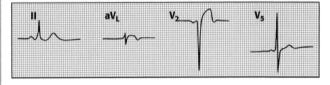

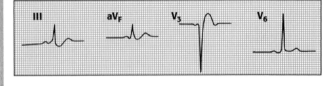

Recognizing an inferior-wall MI

This 12-lead electrocardiogram shows the characteristic changes of an inferior-wall myocardial infarction (MI). In leads II, III, and aV$_F$, note the T-wave inversion, ST-segment elevation, and pathologic Q waves. In leads I and aV$_L$, note the slight ST-segment depression—a reciprocal change.

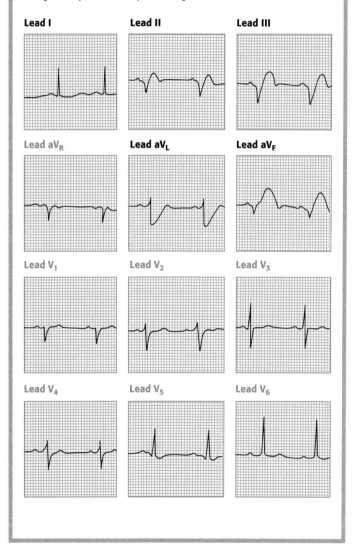

Recognizing a lateral-wall MI

This 12-lead electrocardiogram shows typical characteristics of a lateral-wall myocardial infarction (MI). Note the ST-segment elevation in leads I, aV$_L$, V$_5$, and V$_6$.

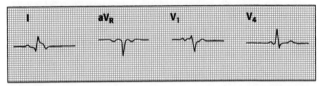

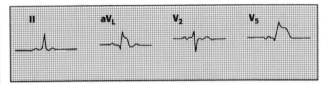

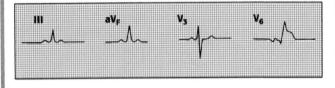

Recognizing a right–ventricular-wall MI

This 12-lead electrocardiogram shows typical traits of a right–ventricular-wall myocardial infarction (MI). Note the ST-segment elevation in the right precordial chest leads V_{4R}, V_{5R}, and V_{6R}. Pathologic Q waves would also appear in leads V_{4R}, V_{5R}, and V_{6R}.

Left-side leads   **Right-side leads**

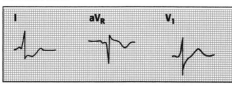

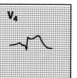

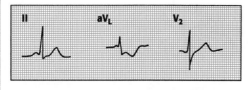

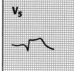

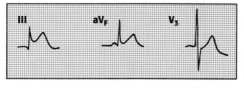

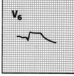

Reciprocal changes in MI

Ischemia, injury, and infarction—the three I's of myocardial infarction (MI)—produce characteristic electrocardiogram (ECG) changes. The changes shown by leads that reflect electrical activity in damaged areas are shown to the right of the illustration below.

Reciprocal leads, those opposite the damaged area, show opposing ECG changes, as shown to the left of the illustration.

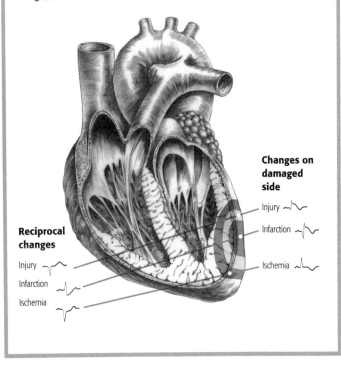

Changes on damaged side

Injury

Infarction

Ischemia

Reciprocal changes

Injury

Infarction

Ischemia

Pericarditis

◆ Inflammation of the pericardium, the fibroserous sac that envelops the heart.
◆ Acute pericarditis:
  – May be fibrinous or effusive.
  – May include purulent, serous, or hemorrhagic exudates.
◆ Chronic pericarditis:
  – Causes dense fibrous thickening of the pericardium.

Recognizing pericarditis

Electrocardiogram changes in acute pericarditis evolve through two stages.

◆ Stage 1: Diffuse ST-segment elevations of 1 to 2 mm in most limb leads and most precordial leads reflect the inflammatory process. Upright T waves appear in most leads. The ST-segment and T-wave changes are typically seen in leads I, II, III, aV_L, aV_F, and V_2 through V_6.

◆ Stage 2: As pericarditis resolves, the ST-segment elevation and accompanying T-wave inversion resolves in most leads.

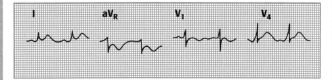

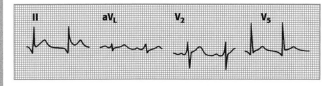

Comparing MI with acute pericarditis

Myocardial infarction (MI) and acute pericarditis each cause ST-segment elevation on an electrocardiogram (ECG). However, the ST segment and T wave (shaded areas) on an MI waveform are quite different from those on a pericarditis waveform, as shown below.

Also, because pericarditis involves the surrounding pericardium, several leads will show ST-segment and T-wave changes (typically leads I, II, III, aV_L, aV_F, and V_2 through V_6). In an MI, only leads reflecting the area of infarction will show the characteristic changes.

Myocardial infarction

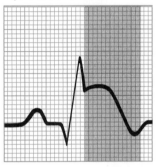

Acute pericarditis

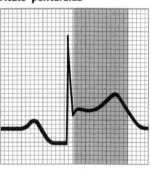

CAUSES

♦ Autoimmune disorders.
♦ Bacterial, fungal, or viral disorders.
♦ Complications of cardiac injury (MI, cardiotomy).
♦ High-dose radiation therapy to the chest.
♦ Rheumatic fever.

SIGNS AND SYMPTOMS

◆ Acute pericarditis:
  – Arrhythmias.
  – Chest pain that typically worsens with deep inspiration and improves when the patient sits up and leans forward.
  – Chills.
  – Diaphoresis.
  – Dyspnea.
  – Fever.
  – Pericardial friction rub.
◆ Chronic pericarditis:
  – Symptoms similar to those of chronic right-sided heart failure (edema, ascites, and hepatomegaly).
  – Palpable, sometimes audible, sharp knock or rub in early diastole, when the rapidly filling ventricle touches the unexpansive pericardium.

 Interventions

◆ Identification and treatment of the underlying cause.
◆ *Acute pericarditis:* Bed rest and corticosteroids or nonsteroidal anti-inflammatory drugs to relieve pain and inflammation.
◆ *Infectious pericarditis:* Antibiotics.
◆ *Cardiac tamponade:* Pericardiocentesis.
◆ *Constrictive pericarditis:* Complete pericardiectomy.

Left ventricular hypertrophy

◆ Known by a thickened left ventricular wall.
◆ Results from conditions that cause chronically increased pressure in the ventricle.
◆ May lead to left-sided heart failure and subsequent changes:
  – Increased left atrial pressure.
  – Pulmonary vascular congestion.
  – Pulmonary arterial hypertension.
◆ May decrease coronary artery perfusion, causing an MI.
◆ May alter the papillary muscle, causing mitral insufficiency.

Recognizing left ventricular hypertrophy

Left ventricular hypertrophy (LVH) can lead to heart failure or myocardial infarction. The rhythm strips shown here illustrate key electrocardiogram changes of LVH as they occur in selected leads: a large S wave (shaded area below left) in V_1 and a large R wave (shaded area below right) in V_5. If the depth (in mm) of the S wave in V_1 added to the height (in mm) of the R wave in V_5 exceeds 35 mm, then the patient has left ventricular hypertrophy.

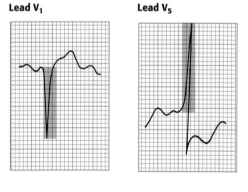

Lead V_1 Lead V_5

CAUSES

- ◆ Aortic stenosis or insufficiency.
- ◆ Cardiomyopathy.
- ◆ Mitral insufficiency.
- ◆ Systemic hypertension (most common).

SIGNS AND SYMPTOMS

- ◆ Related to the underlying disorder.

 Interventions

◆ Interventions focus on proper management of the underlying disorder, such as hypertension.

Bundle-branch block

♦ A potential complication of MI.
♦ QRS complex more than 0.12 second.
♦ Abnormal impulse conduction through the left or right bundle branch.
♦ Impulse pathway down the unaffected bundle branch and from one myocardial cell to the next to depolarize the ventricle.
♦ Prolonged ventricular depolarization because cell-to-cell conduction progresses much more slowly than along the specialized cells of the conduction system.
♦ May be treated with a temporary pacemaker.
♦ May be monitored to detect progression to a more complete block.

Understanding right bundle-branch block

In right bundle-branch block, the initial impulse activates the interventricular septum from left to right, just as in normal activation (arrow 1). Next, the left bundle branch activates the left ventricle (arrow 2). The impulse then crosses the interventricular septum to activate the right ventricle (arrow 3).

In this disorder, the QRS complex exceeds 0.12 second and has a different configuration, sometimes resembling rabbit ears or the letter "M." Septal depolarization isn't affected in lead V_1, so the initial small R wave remains.

The R wave is followed by an S wave, which represents left ventricular depolarization, and a tall R wave (called R prime, or R'), which represents late right ventricular depolarization. The T wave is negative in this lead; however, the negative deflection is called a secondary T-wave change and isn't clinically significant.

The opposite occurs in lead V_6. A small Q wave is followed by depolarization of the left ventricle, which produces a tall R wave. Depolarization of the right ventricle then causes a broad S wave. In lead V_6, the T wave should be positive.

Right bundle-branch block occurs with such conditions as anterior-wall myocardial infarction, coronary artery disease, and pulmonary embolism. However, it also may occur without cardiac disease. If it develops as the patient's heart rate increases, it's known as rate-related right bundle-branch block.

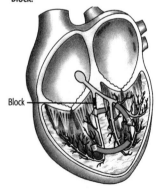

Block

Recognizing right bundle-branch block

This 12-lead electrocardiogram shows the characteristic changes of right bundle-branch block. In lead V_1, note the rsR′ pattern and T-wave inversion. In lead V_6, see the widened S wave and the upright T wave. Also note the prolonged QRS complexes.

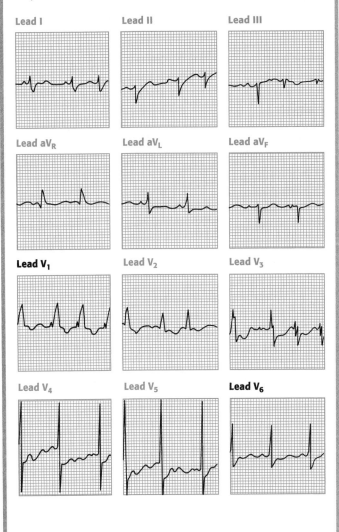

Understanding left bundle-branch block

In left bundle-branch block, an impulse first travels down the right bundle branch (arrow 1). Then it activates the interventricular septum from right to left (arrow 2), the opposite of normal activation. Finally, the impulse activates the left ventricle (arrow 3).

On an electrocardiogram, the QRS complex exceeds 0.12 second because the ventricles are activated sequentially, not simultaneously. As the wave of depolarization spreads from the right ventricle to the left, a wide S wave appears in lead V₁ with a positive T wave. The S wave may be preceded by a Q wave or a small R wave.

In lead V₆, no initial Q wave occurs. A tall, notched R wave, or a slurred one, appears as the impulse spreads from right to left. This initial positive deflection is a sign of left bundle-branch block. The T wave is negative.

Left bundle-branch block never occurs normally. It usually results from hypertensive heart disease, aortic stenosis, degenerative changes of the conduction system, or coronary artery disease. If it accompanies an anterior- wall myocardial infarction and results in complete heart block, the patient may need a pacemaker.

Keep in mind that it may be difficult to differentiate between bundle-branch block and Wolff-Parkinson-White (WPW) syndrome. Whenever you spot what seems to be bundle-branch block, check for WPW syndrome as well.

Block

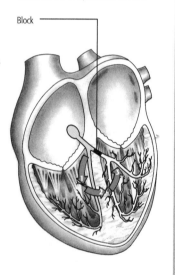

Recognizing left bundle-branch block

This 12-lead electrocardiogram shows characteristic changes of a left bundle-branch block. All leads have prolonged QRS complexes. In lead V_1, note the QS wave pattern. In lead V_6, you can see the slurred R wave and T-wave inversion. The elevated ST segments and upright T waves in leads V_1 to V_4 are also common in this condition.

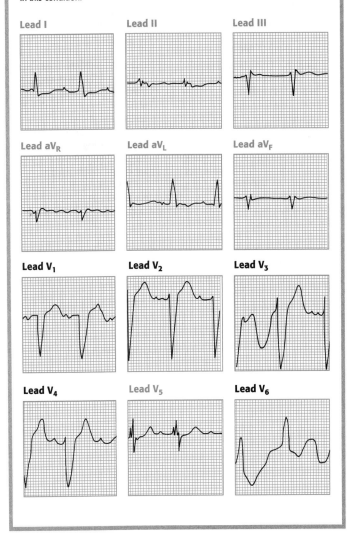

Lead I   Lead II   Lead III

Lead aV_R Lead aV_L Lead aV_F

Lead V_1 Lead V_2 Lead V_3

Lead V_4 Lead V_5 Lead V_6

Distinguishing bundle-branch block from Wolff-Parkinson-White syndrome

Wolff-Parkinson-White (WPW) syndrome is a common type of preexcitation syndrome, an abnormal condition in which electrical impulses enter the ventricles from the atria using an accessory pathway that bypasses the atrioventricular (AV) junction. This results in a short PR interval and a wide QRS complex with an initial slurring of the upward slope of the QRS complex, called a delta wave. Because the delta wave prolongs the QRS complex, it may be confused with a bundle-branch block.

Bundle-branch block

♦ Carefully examine the QRS complex, noting which part of the complex is widened. A bundle-branch block involves defective conduction of electrical impulses through the right or left bundle branch from the bundle of His to the Purkinje network.

♦ This conduction disturbance results either in an overall increase in QRS duration or a widening of the last part of the QRS complex with the initial part of the QRS complex commonly appearing normal.

♦ Carefully examine the 12-lead electrocardiogram (ECG). With a bundle-branch block, the prolonged duration of the QRS complexes usually will be consistent in all leads.

♦ Measure the PR interval. A bundle-branch block has no effect on the PR interval, so the PR intervals typically are normal. Keep in mind, though, that if the patient has an AV conduction defect, such as first-degree AV block, the PR interval will be prolonged.

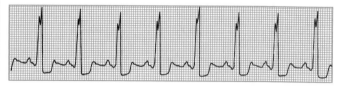

Wolff-Parkinson-White syndrome

◆ A delta wave occurs at the beginning of the QRS complex, usually causing a distinctive slurring or hump in its initial slope. A delta wave isn't present in bundle-branch block.

◆ On the 12-lead ECG, the delta wave will be most pronounced in the leads looking at the part of the heart where the accessory pathway is located.

◆ The delta wave shortens the PR interval in WPW syndrome.

Short PR interval   Delta wave

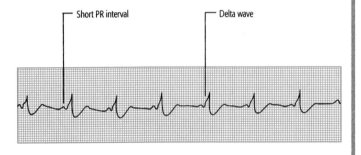

Conduction in Wolff-Parkinson-White syndrome

Electrical impulses don't always follow normal conduction pathways in the heart. In preexcitation syndromes, electrical impulses enter the ventricles from the atria through an accessory pathway that bypasses the atrioventricular junction. Wolff-Parkinson-White (WPW) syndrome is a common type of preexcitation syndrome.

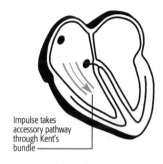

Impulse takes accessory pathway through Kent's bundle

WPW syndrome commonly occurs in young children and in adults ages 20 to 35. The syndrome causes the PR interval to shorten and the QRS complex to lengthen as a result of a delta wave. Delta waves, which occur just before normal ventricular depolarization in WPW syndrome, are produced as a result of premature depolarization (preexcitation) of a portion of the ventricles.

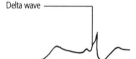

Delta wave

WPW syndrome is clinically significant because the accessory pathway — in this case, Kent's bundle — may result in paroxysmal tachyarrhythmias by reentry and rapid conduction mechanisms.

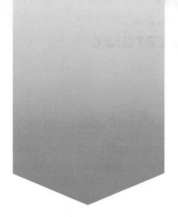

Appendices

Selected references

Index

Quick guide to cardiac arrhythmias

Here's an outline of many common cardiac arrhythmias and their features, causes, and treatments. Use a normal electrocardiogram strip, if available, to compare normal cardiac rhythm configurations with the rhythm strips shown here. Characteristics of normal sinus rhythm include the following:

- Ventricular and atrial rates of 60 to 100 beats/minute.
- Regular and uniform QRS complexes and P waves.
- PR interval of 0.12 to 0.20 second.

- QRS duration < 0.12 second.
- Identical atrial and ventricular rates, with constant PR intervals.

Arrhythmia and features

Sinus tachycardia

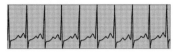

- Atrial and ventricular rhythms regular.
- Rate > 100 beats/minute; rarely, > 160 beats/minute.
- Normal P waves preceding each QRS complex.

Sinus bradycardia

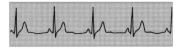

- Atrial and ventricular rhythms regular.
- Rate < 60 beats/minute.
- Normal P waves preceding each QRS complex.

Causes	Treatment
◆ Normal physiologic response to fever, exercise, anxiety, pain, dehydration; may also accompany shock, left-sided heart failure, cardiac tamponade, hyperthyroidism, anemia, hypovolemia, pulmonary embolism, and anterior-wall myocardial infarction (MI).	◆ Correction of underlying cause.
	◆ Beta blockers or calcium channel blocker.
◆ May also occur with atropine, epinephrine, isoproterenol, quinidine, caffeine, alcohol, cocaine, amphetamine, and nicotine use.	
◆ Normal in well-conditioned heart, as in an athlete.	◆ Correction of underlying cause.
◆ Increased intracranial pressure; increased vagal tone from straining during defecation, vomiting, intubation, or mechanical ventilation; sick sinus syndrome; hypothyroidism; and inferior-wall MI.	◆ For low cardiac output, dizziness, weakness, altered level of consciousness, or low blood pressure; advanced cardiac life support (ACLS) protocol for administration of atropine.
◆ May also occur with anticholinesterase, beta blocker, digoxin, and morphine use.	◆ Temporary or permanent pacemaker.
	◆ Dopamine or epinephrine infusion.

Arrhythmia and features

Paroxysmal supraventricular tachycardia

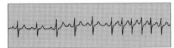

- ◆ Atrial and ventricular rhythms regular.
- ◆ Heart rate > 160 beats/minute; rarely exceeds 250 beats/minute.
- ◆ P waves regular but aberrant; difficult to differentiate from preceding T waves.
- ◆ P waves preceding each QRS complex.
- ◆ Sudden onset and termination of arrhythmia.

Atrial flutter

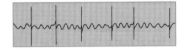

- ◆ Atrial rhythm regular; rate 250 to 400 beats/minute.
- ◆ Ventricular rate variable, depending on degree of AV block (usually 60 to 100 beats/minute).
- ◆ No P waves; atrial activity appears as flutter waves (F waves); sawtooth configuration common in lead II.
- ◆ QRS complexes are uniform in shape but often irregular in rhythm.

Atrial fibrillation

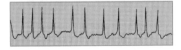

- ◆ Atrial rhythm grossly irregular; rate > 400 beats/minute.
- ◆ Ventricular rhythm grossly irregular.
- ◆ QRS complexes of uniform configuration and duration.
- ◆ PR interval indiscernible.
- ◆ No P waves; atrial activity appears as erratic, irregular, baseline fibrillatory waves (f waves).

Causes	**Treatment**
◆ Intrinsic abnormality of atrioventricular (AV) conduction system. ◆ Physical or psychological stress, hypoxia, hypokalemia, cardiomyopathy, congenital heart disease, MI, valvular disease, Wolff-Parkinson-White syndrome, cor pulmonale, hyperthyroidism, and systemic hypertension. ◆ Digoxin toxicity; use of caffeine, marijuana, or central nervous system stimulants.	◆ If patient is unstable, immediate cardioversion. ◆ If patient is stable, vagal stimulation, Valsalva's maneuver, and carotid sinus massage or adenosine. ◆ If cardiac function is preserved, treatment priority: calcium channel blocker, beta blocker, digoxin, and cardioversion; then consider procainamide, or amiodarone if each preceding treatment is ineffective in rhythm conversion. ◆ If the ejection fraction is less than 40% or if the patient is in heart failure, treatment order: digoxin, amiodarone, and then diltiazem.
◆ Heart failure, tricuspid or mitral valve disease, pulmonary embolism, cor pulmonale, inferior-wall MI, and pericarditis. ◆ Digoxin toxicity.	◆ If patient is unstable with a ventricular rate > 150 beats/minute, immediate cardioversion. ◆ If patient is stable, follow ACLS protocol for cardioversion and drug therapy, which may include calcium channel blockers, beta blockers, amiodarone, or digoxin. ◆ Anticoagulation therapy may also be needed. ◆ Radio frequency ablation to control rhythm.
◆ Heart failure, chronic obstructive pulmonary disease, thyrotoxicosis, constrictive pericarditis, ischemic heart disease, sepsis, pulmonary embolus, rheumatic heart disease, hypertension, mitral stenosis, atrial irritation, or complication of coronary bypass or valve replacement surgery. ◆ Nifedipine and digoxin use.	◆ If patient is unstable with a ventricular rate > 150 beats/minute, immediate cardioversion. ◆ If patient is stable, follow ACLS protocol and drug therapy, which may include calcium channel blockers, beta blockers, amiodarone, or digoxin. ◆ Anticoagulation therapy may also be needed. ◆ In some patients with refractory atrial fibrillation uncontrolled by drugs, radio frequency catheter ablation.

Arrhythmia and features

Junctional rhythm

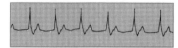

- ◆ Atrial and ventricular rhythms regular; atrial rate 40 to 60 beats/minute; ventricular rate usually 40 to 60 beats/minute (60 to 100 beats/minute is accelerated junctional rhythm).
- ◆ P waves preceding, hidden within (absent), or after QRS complex; usually inverted if visible.
- ◆ PR interval (when present) < 0.12 second.
- ◆ QRS complex configuration and duration normal, except in aberrant conduction.

First-degree AV block

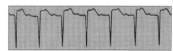

- ◆ Atrial and ventricular rhythms regular.
- ◆ PR interval > 0.20 second.
- ◆ P wave precedes QRS complex.
- ◆ QRS complex normal.

Second-degree AV block
Mobitz I (Wenckebach)

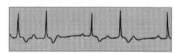

- ◆ Atrial rhythm regular.
- ◆ Ventricular rhythm irregular.
- ◆ Atrial rate exceeds ventricular rate.
- ◆ PR interval progressively longer with each cycle until QRS complex disappears (dropped beat); PR interval shorter after dropped beat.

Second-degree AV block
Mobitz II

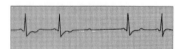

- ◆ Atrial rhythm regular.
- ◆ Ventricular rhythm regular or irregular, with varying degree of block.
- ◆ PR interval constant for conducted beats.
- ◆ P waves normal size and shape, but some aren't followed by a QRS complex.

Causes	Treatment

- ◆ Inferior-wall MI or ischemia, hypoxia, vagal stimulation, and sick sinus syndrome.
- ◆ Acute rheumatic fever.
- ◆ Valve surgery.
- ◆ Digoxin toxicity.

- ◆ Correction of underlying cause.
- ◆ Atropine for symptomatic slow rate.
- ◆ Pacemaker insertion if patient doesn't respond to drugs.
- ◆ Discontinuation of digoxin if appropriate.

- ◆ May be seen in healthy persons.
- ◆ Inferior-wall MI or ischemia, hypothyroidism, hypokalemia, and hyperkalemia.
- ◆ Digoxin toxicity; use of quinidine, procainamide, beta blockers, calcium channel blockers, or amiodarone.

- ◆ Correction of underlying cause.
- ◆ Possibly atropine if severe symptomatic bradycardia develops.
- ◆ Cautious use of digoxin, calcium channel blockers, and beta blockers.

- ◆ Inferior-wall MI, cardiac surgery, acute rheumatic fever, and vagal stimulation.
- ◆ Digoxin toxicity; use of propranolol, quinidine, or procainamide.

- ◆ Treatment of underlying cause.
- ◆ Atropine or temporary pacemaker for symptomatic bradycardia.
- ◆ Discontinuation of digoxin if appropriate.

- ◆ Severe coronary artery disease, anterior-wall MI, and acute myocarditis.
- ◆ Digoxin toxicity.

- ◆ Temporary or permanent pacemaker.
- ◆ Atropine, dopamine, or epinephrine for a symptomatic bradycardia.
- ◆ Discontinuation of digoxin if appropriate.

Arrhythmia and features

Third-degree AV block
(complete heart block)

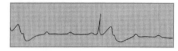

- ◆ Atrial rhythm regular.
- ◆ Ventricular rhythm regular and rate slower than atrial rate.
- ◆ No relation between P waves and QRS complexes.
- ◆ No constant PR interval.
- ◆ QRS duration normal (junctional pacemaker) or wide and bizarre (ventricular pacemaker).

Premature ventricular contraction (PVC)

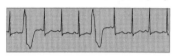

- ◆ Atrial rhythm regular.
- ◆ Ventricular rhythm irregular.
- ◆ QRS complex premature, usually followed by a complete compensatory pause.
- ◆ QRS complex wide and distorted, usually > 0.12 second.
- ◆ Premature QRS complexes occurring alone, in pairs, or in threes, alternating with normal beats; focus from one or more sites.
- ◆ Ominous when clustered, multifocal, with R-wave-on-T pattern.

Causes	Treatment

◆ Inferior- or anterior-wall MI, congenital abnormality, rheumatic fever, hypoxia, postoperative complication of mitral valve replacement, postprocedure complication of radiofrequency ablation in or near AV nodal tissue, Lev's disease (fibrosis and calcification that spreads from cardiac structures to the conductive tissue), and Lenégre's disease (conductive tissue fibrosis).
◆ Digoxin toxicity.

◆ Atropine, dopamine, or epinephrine for symptomatic bradycardia.
◆ Temporary or permanent pacemaker.

◆ Heart failure; old or acute MI, ischemia, or contusion; myocardial irritation by ventricular catheter or a pacemaker; hypercapnia; hypokalemia; hypocalcemia; and hypomagnesemia.
◆ Drug toxicity (digoxin, aminophylline, tricyclic antidepressants, beta blockers, isoproterenol, or dopamine).
◆ Caffeine, tobacco, or alcohol use.
◆ Psychological stress, anxiety, pain, or exercise.

◆ If warranted, procainamide, amiodarone, or lidocaine I.V.
◆ Treatment of underlying cause.
◆ Discontinuation of drug causing toxicity.
◆ Potassium chloride I.V. if PVC induced by hypokalemia.
◆ Magnesium sulfate I.V. if PVC induced by hypomagnesemia.

Arrhythmia and features

Ventricular tachycardia

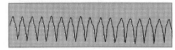

- ◆ Ventricular rate 100 to 220 beats/minute, rhythm usually regular.
- ◆ QRS complexes wide, bizarre, and independent of P waves.
- ◆ P waves not discernible.
- ◆ May start and stop suddenly.

Ventricular fibrillation

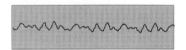

- ◆ Ventricular rhythm and rate chaotic and rapid.
- ◆ QRS complexes wide and irregular; no visible P waves.

Causes	Treatment

- ◆ Myocardial ischemia, MI, or aneurysm; coronary artery disease; rheumatic heart disease; mitral valve prolapse; heart failure; cardiomyopathy; ventricular catheters; hypokalemia; hypercalcemia; hypomagnesemia; and pulmonary embolism.
- ◆ Digoxin, procainamde, epinephrine, or quinidine toxicity.
- ◆ Anxiety.

- ◆ With pulse: If hemodynamically stable with monomorphic QRS complexes, administration of procainamide, sotalol, amiodarone, or lidocaine (follow ACLS protocol); if drugs are ineffective, cardioversion.
- ◆ If polymorphic QRS complexes and normal QT interval, administer beta blockers, lidocaine, amiodarone, procainamide, or sotalol (follow ACLS protocol); if drug is unsuccessful, cardioversion.
- ◆ If polymorphic QRS and QT interval is prolonged, magnesium I.V., and then overdrive pacing if rhythm persists; may also administer isoproterenol, phenytoin, or lidocaine.
- ◆ Pulseless: Start CPR; follow ACLS protocol for defibrillation, endotracheal (ET) intubation, and administration of epinephrine or vasopressin, followed by amiodarone or lidocaine and, if ineffective, magnesium sulfate or procainamide.
- ◆ Implantable cardioverter-defibrillator (ICD) if recurrent ventricular tachycardia.

- ◆ Myocardial ischemia, MI, untreated ventricular tachycardia, R-on-T phenomenon, hypokalemia, hyperkalemia, hypercalcemia, hypoxemia, alkalosis, electric shock, and hypothermia.
- ◆ Digoxin, epinephrine, or quinidine toxicity.

- ◆ CPR; follow ACLS protocol for defibrillation, ET intubation, and administration of epinephrine or vasopressin, amiodarone, or lidocaine and, if ineffective, magnesium sulfate or procainamide.
- ◆ ICD if risk for recurrent ventricular fibrillation.

Arrhythmia and features

Asystole

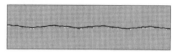

◆ No atrial or ventricular rate or rhythm.
◆ No discernible P waves, QRS complexes, or T waves.

Causes	**Treatment**
◆ Myocardial ischemia, MI, aortic valve disease, heart failure, hypoxia, hypokalemia, severe acidosis, electric shock, ventricular arrhythmia, AV block, pulmonary embolism, heart rupture, cardiac tamponade, hyperkalemia, and electromechanical dissociation.	◆ Continue CPR, follow ACLS protocol for ET intubation, temporary pacing, and administration of epinephrine and atropine.
◆ Cocaine overdose.	

Cardiac drug overview

Drug	Action	Indications
adenosine (Adenocard)	◆ Slows conduction through the atrioventricular (AV) node.	Paroxysmal supraventricular tachycardia (PSVT), including Wolff-Parkinson-White syndrome.
amiodarone hydrochloride (Cordarone)	◆ Blocks sodium channels at rapid pacing frequencies.	Life-threatening ventricular arrhythmias, such as recurrent ventricular fibrillation and recurrent, hemodynamically unstable ventricular tachycardia.
calcium channel blockers (amlodipine, bepridil hydrochloride, diltiazem hydrochloride, felodipine, isradipine, nicardipine hydrochloride, nifedipine, nimodipine, nisoldipine, verapamil)	◆ Inhibit influx of calcium through the cell membrane, resulting in a depression of automaticity and conduction velocity in smooth and cardiac muscles. ◆ Different degrees of selectivity on vascular smooth muscle, myocardium, and conduction and pacemaker tissues.	Vary for each drug.

Adverse effects	**Special considerations**
◆ Chest pain. ◆ Dyspnea. ◆ Flushing. ◆ Transient sinus bradycardia and ventricular ectopy.	◆ Use cautiously in patients with denervated transplanted hearts. ◆ A brief period of asystole (up to 15 seconds) may occur after rapid administration. ◆ Rapidly follow each dose with a 20-ml saline flush. ◆ Don't administer through a central line because a more prolonged asystole may result.
◆ Pulmonary fibrosis. ◆ Bradycardia. ◆ Exacerbation of arrhythmia. ◆ Fever. ◆ Heart failure. ◆ Nausea and vomiting. ◆ Hepatotoxicity. ◆ Hypotension. ◆ Ophthalmic abnormalities: Corneal microdeposits. ◆ Hypothyroidism. ◆ Hyperthyroidism. ◆ Photosensitivity and skin discoloration.	◆ Closely monitor the patient during loading phase. ◆ Administer doses with meals. ◆ If the patient needs a dosage adjustment, monitor him for an extended time because of the drug's long and variable half-life and the difficulty in predicting the time needed to achieve new steady-state plasma drug level. ◆ Monitor need to adjust dose of digoxin or warfarin.
◆ Adverse effects vary among calcium channel blockers; refer to individual drug.	◆ Hypertensive patients treated with calcium channel blockers have a higher risk of heart attack than patients treated with diuretics or beta blockers. ◆ Abrupt withdrawal may result in increased frequency and duration of chest pain. ◆ Monitor cardiac and respiratory function. ◆ Don't use for a patient with Wolff-Parkinson-White syndrome.

Drug	Action	Indications
cardiac glycosides (digoxin)	◆ Increase force and velocity of myocardial contraction by increasing refractory period of AV node and increasing total peripheral resistance. ◆ Digitoxin: slower onset and more potent than digoxin.	Slow heart rate in sinus tachycardia from heart failure and control of rapid ventricular contraction rate in patients with atrial fibrillation or flutter.
disopyramide phosphate (Norpace)	◆ Decreases rate of diastolic depolarization and upstroke velocity; increases action potential duration; prolongs refractory period.	Life-threatening ventricular arrhythmias such as sustained ventricular tachycardia.
dofetilide (Tikosyn)	◆ Blocks cardiac potassium channels; increases duration of action potential by delaying repolarization.	Maintains sinus rhythm in patients with chronic atrial fibrillation or atrial flutter.
flecainide acetate (Tambocor)	◆ Decreases single and multiple premature ventricular contractions (PVCs); reduces incidence of ventricular tachycardia. ◆ Effect results from a local anesthetic action, especially on the His-Purkinje system in the ventricle.	Sustained ventricular tachycardia.
ibutilide fumarate (Corvert)	◆ Delays repolarization by activating slow, inward current (mostly sodium), which results in prolonged duration of atrial and ventricular action potential and refractoriness.	Rapid conversion of recent-onset atrial fibrillation or atrial flutter.

Adverse effects	**Special considerations**
◆ AV block. ◆ Bradycardia. ◆ Headaches. ◆ Hypokalemia. ◆ Nausea and vomiting. ◆ Visual disturbances.	◆ Cardiac glycosides are extremely toxic, with a narrow margin of safety between therapeutic range and toxicity. ◆ Vomiting is usually an early sign of drug toxicity. ◆ Discontinue cardiac glycosides as ordered if patient's pulse rate falls below 60 beats/minute.
◆ Chest pain. ◆ First-degree AV block. ◆ Hypotension. ◆ Nausea. ◆ Long QT interval. ◆ Prolonged QRS.	◆ Disopyramide increases risk of death in patients with non–life-threatening ventricular arrhythmias. ◆ Use cautiously in patients with Wolff-Parkinson-White syndrome or bundle-branch block.
◆ Torsades de pointes. ◆ Chest pain. ◆ Headache.	◆ Don't use if baseline QTc is greater than 440 msec, if baseline heart rate is less than 50 beats/minute, or if severe renal impairment exists. ◆ Must be initiated by cardiologist, with continuous ECG monitoring for at least 3 days. ◆ Don't use with cimetidine, verapamil, ketoconazole, or trimethoprim.
◆ Dizziness. ◆ Dyspnea. ◆ Headache. ◆ Nausea. ◆ Ventricular arrhythmias (new or worsened). ◆ Visual disturbances.	◆ Contraindicated in patients with structural heart disease. ◆ Periodically monitor trough plasma levels because 40% is bound to plasma protein. ◆ Increase dosage as ordered at intervals of more than 4 days in renal patients.
◆ Nausea. ◆ Headache. ◆ Torsades de pointes. ◆ Worsening ventricular tachycardia. ◆ Prolonged QT interval. ◆ Hypotension.	◆ Stop drug infusion as ordered when arrhythmia stops, if ventricular tachycardia occurs, or if QT interval becomes markedly prolonged. ◆ Perform continuous ECG monitoring for at least 4 hours after dose is completed because of proarrhythmic risk. ◆ Check potassium and magnesium levels and correct before giving drug.

Drug	Action	Indications
lidocaine hydrochloride (Xylocaine)	◆ Shortens the refractory period and suppresses the automaticity of ectopic foci without affecting conduction of impulses through cardiac tissue.	Acute ventricular arrhythmias.
moricizine hydrochloride (Ethmozine)	◆ Shortens phase II and III repolarization, leading to decreased duration of the action potential and an effective refractory period.	Life-threatening ventricular arrhythmias such as sustained ventricular tachycardia.
phenytoin sodium (Dilantin)	◆ Increases the electrical stimulation threshold of heart muscle.	PVCs and tachycardia, especially arrhythmias from digoxin overdose.
procainamide hydrochloride (Procanbid, Pronestyl)	◆ Produces a direct cardiac effect to prolong the refractory period of the atria and (to a lesser extent) the His-Purkinje system and the ventricles.	Potentially life-threatening ventricular arrhythmias when benefits of treatment clearly outweigh risks.
propafenone hydrochloride (Rythmol)	◆ Reduces upstroke velocity of monophasic action potential. ◆ Reduces fast, inward current carried by sodium ions in Purkinje fibers. ◆ Increases diastolic excitability threshold. ◆ Prolongs effective refractory period.	Life-threatening ventricular arrhythmias such as ventricular tachycardia when benefits of treatment outweigh risk.

Adverse effects	**Special considerations**
◆ Dizziness. ◆ Hallucinations. ◆ Nervousness. ◆ Tachycardia. ◆ Tachypnea. ◆ Seizures.	◆ Lidocaine doesn't affect blood pressure, cardiac output, or myocardial contractility. ◆ Lidocaine is ineffective against atrial arrhythmias. ◆ Contraindicated in second- or third-degree AV block without pacing support. ◆ Reduce drug dosage as ordered in patients with heart failure or liver disease. ◆ Monitor patient closely for CNS changes.
◆ Bradycardia. ◆ Dizziness. ◆ Headache. ◆ Nausea. ◆ Sustained ventricular tachycardia.	◆ Use cautiously in patients with sick sinus syndrome because of the possibility of sinus bradycardia, sinus pause, or sinus arrest. ◆ The patient should be hospitalized for initial dosing. ◆ Give before meals because food delays rate of absorption.
◆ Ataxia. ◆ Drowsiness. ◆ Hepatocellular necrosis (fatal). ◆ Hypotension. ◆ Nervousness.	◆ Phenytoin is also used for treatment of chronic epilepsy. ◆ Monitor serum levels. ◆ Abrupt withdrawal may cause status epilepticus. ◆ Use with extreme caution in patients with hypotension or severe myocardial insufficiency.
◆ Hypotension. ◆ Diarrhea. ◆ Dizziness. ◆ Liver failure. ◆ Lupus erythematosus-like syndrome. ◆ Nausea and vomiting. ◆ Heart block. ◆ Agranulocytosis.	◆ Procainamide increases risk of death in patients with non–life-threatening arrhythmias. ◆ Use with caution in patients with liver or kidney dysfunction. ◆ Tell patient not to crush or break extended-release tablets.
◆ Constipation. ◆ Dizziness. ◆ AV block. ◆ Headache. ◆ Nausea and vomiting. ◆ Unusual taste. ◆ Ventricular tachycardia.	◆ Monitor liver and renal function studies. ◆ Report any significant widening of QRS complex and any evidence of second- or third-degree AV block. ◆ Increase dosage more gradually as ordered in elderly patients and patients with previous myocardial damage.

Drug	Action	Indications
propranolol hydrochloride (Inderal)	◆ Antiarrhythmic action results from beta-adrenergic receptor blockade as well as a direct membrane stabilization action on cardiac cells.	Cardiac arrhythmias, such as ventricular tachycardias, supra-ventricular arrhyth-mias, and PVCs.
quinidine sulfate (Quinidex)	◆ Reduces excitability of the heart and depresses conduc-tion velocity and contractility. ◆ Prolongs refractory period and increases conduction time.	Atrial flutter or fibril-lation, paroxysmal atrial tachycardia, paroxysmal AV junc-tional rhythm, and paroxysmal ventricu-lar tachycardia.
sotalol (Betapace)	◆ Antiarrhythmic with beta-blocking effects and prolonga-tion of the action potential. ◆ Slows AV nodal conduction and increases AV nodal refrac-toriness.	Life-threatening ven-tricular arrhythmias. Maintains sinus rhythm in patients with history of symp-tomatic atrial fibrilla-tion or atrial flutter.

Adverse effects	**Special considerations**
◆ Bradycardia. ◆ Heart failure. ◆ Hypotension. ◆ Light-headedness. ◆ Nausea and vomiting.	◆ Propranolol is also used for treatment of hypertension, angina pectoris, and MI. ◆ Dosages may differ for hypertension, angina, or MI. ◆ If signs of serious myocardial depression occur, slowly infuse I.V. isoproterenol (Isuprel).
◆ Angina-like pain. ◆ Complete AV block. ◆ Diarrhea. ◆ Headache. ◆ Hypotension. ◆ Light-headedness. ◆ Torsades de pointes.	◆ Notify physician at once if widening QRS complex or increased AV block becomes apparent. ◆ Use with extreme caution in patients who develop a sudden change in blood pressure. ◆ Give with food to minimize GI effects.
◆ Bradycardia. ◆ Chest pain. ◆ Dizziness. ◆ Fatigue. ◆ Palpitations. ◆ QT prolongation.	◆ Contraindicated in patients with bronchial asthma, sinus bradycardia, or second- or third-degree AV block without a pacemaker. ◆ Perform ECG monitoring for at least 3 days when therapy starts. ◆ Adjust dosage in renally impaired patients. ◆ Assess patient for QTc prolongation. ◆ Administer drug when patient has an empty stomach.

Best monitoring leads

The best monitoring lead is determined by the patient's medical condition and by the arrhythmias most likely to occur. Most bedside monitoring systems allow for simultaneous monitoring of two leads such as lead II with V_1 or MCL_1.

Lead II or the best lead that clearly shows P waves and the QRS complex may be used for sinus node arrhythmias, premature atrial contractions, and atrioventricular block

The precordial leads V_1 and V_6 or the bipolar leads MCL_1 and MCL_6 are the best leads for monitoring rhythms with wide QRS complexes and differentiating ventricular tachycardia from supraventricular tachycardia with aberrancy.

Specific leads may also be used in monitoring patients with acute coronary syndromes.

The table below lists the best leads for monitoring challenging cardiac arrhythmias and special situations such as acute coronary syndromes.

Arrhythmia	Best monitoring leads
◆ Premature atrial contractions	II or lead that shows best P waves
◆ Atrial tachycardia	II, V_1, V_6, MCL_1, MCL_6 (with aberrancy)
◆ Multifocal atrial tachycardia	II, V_1, V_6, MCL_1, MCL_6 (with aberrancy)
◆ Paroxysmal atrial tachycardia	II, V_1, V_6, MCL_1, MCL_6 (with aberrancy)
◆ Atrial flutter	II, III or aV_F
◆ Atrial fibrillation	II (or identified in most leads by fibrillatory waves and irregular R-R)
◆ Premature junctional contractions	II
◆ Junctional escape rhythm	II
◆ Junctional tachycardia	II, V_1, V_6, MCL_1, MCL_6 (with aberrancy)
◆ Premature ventricular contractions	V_1, V_6, MCL_1, MCL_6
◆ Idioventricular rhythm	V_1, V_6, MCL_1, MCL_6
◆ Ventricular tachycardia	V_1, V_6, MCL_1, MCL_6

Arrhythmia	Best monitoring leads
◆ Ventricular fibrillation	Any
◆ Torsades de pointes	Any
◆ Third-degree AV block	II or lead that shows best P waves and QRS complex

Monitoring patients with acute coronary syndromes

Remember that specific leads monitor specific walls of the heart. Here's a quick overview of those leads.

Heart wall	Best monitoring leads
◆ Anterior-wall myocardial infarction (MI)	Lead V_1 or MCL_1
◆ Inferior-wall MI	Lead II, III, aV_F
◆ Lateral-wall MI	Lead V_6 or MCL_6
◆ Septal-wall MI	Lead V_1 or MCL_1

Depolarization-repolarization cycle

The depolarization-repolarization cycle consists of the following phases.

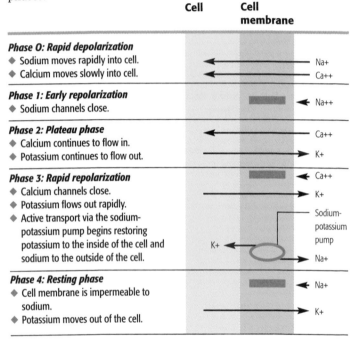

Phase 0: Rapid depolarization
- Sodium moves rapidly into cell.
- Calcium moves slowly into cell.

Phase 1: Early repolarization
- Sodium channels close.

Phase 2: Plateau phase
- Calcium continues to flow in.
- Potassium continues to flow out.

Phase 3: Rapid repolarization
- Calcium channels close.
- Potassium flows out rapidly.
- Active transport via the sodium-potassium pump begins restoring potassium to the inside of the cell and sodium to the outside of the cell.

Phase 4: Resting phase
- Cell membrane is impermeable to sodium.
- Potassium moves out of the cell.

Action potential curves

An action potential curve shows the changes in a cell's electrical charge during the five phases of the depolarization-repolarization cycle. These graphs show electrical changes for pacemaker and nonpacemaker cells.

Action potential curve: Pacemaker cell

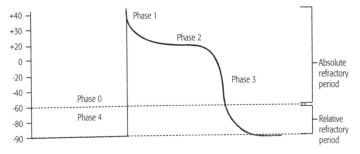

As the graph below shows, the action potential curve for pacemaker cells, such as those in the sinoatrial node, differs from that of other myocardial cells. Pacemaker cells have a resting membrane potential of –60 mV (instead of –90 mV), and they begin to depolarize spontaneously. Called diastolic depolarization, this effect results primarily from calcium and sodium leakage into the cell.

Action potential curve: Nonpacemaker cell

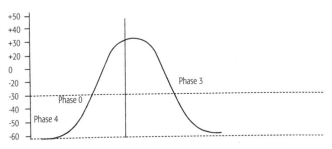

Cardiac conduction system

Specialized fibers propagate electrical impulses throughout the heart's cells, causing the heart to contract. This illustration shows the elements of the cardiac conduction system.

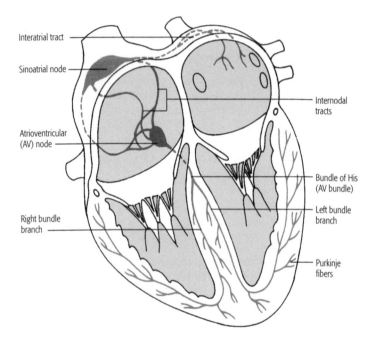

Selected references

Aehlert, B. *ACLS Quick Review Study Guide,* 2nd ed. St. Louis: Mosby–Year Book, Inc., 2002.

Albert, N.M. "Cardiac Resynchronization Therapy through Biventricular Pacing in Patients with Heart Failure and Ventricular Dyssynchrony," *Critical Care Nurse* 23:2-13, June 2003.

Catalano, J. *Guide to ECG Analysis,* 2nd ed. Philadelphia: Lippincott Williams & Wilkins, 2002.

Cosio, F.G., and Delpon, E. "New Antiarrhythmic Drugs for Atrial Flutter and Atrial Fibrillation: A Conceptual Breakthrough at Last?" *Circulation* 105(3):276-78, January 2002.

Dubin, D. Rapid Interpretation of EKGs, 6th ed. Tampa, Fla.: Cover Publishing Company, 2000.

ECG Cards, 4th ed. Philadelphia: Lippincott, Williams & Willkins, 2005.

ECG Interpretation Made Incredibly Easy, 2nd ed. Springhouse, Pa.: Springhouse Corp., 2002.

Faber, T.S., et al. "Impact of Electrocardiogram Recording Format on QT Interval Measurement and QT Dispersion Assessment," *Pacing and Clinical Electrophysiology* 24(12):1739-47, December 2001.

Huikuri, H.V., et al. "Sudden Death Due to Cardiac Arrhythmias," *New England Journal of Medicine* 345(20):1473-82, November 2001.

Landesberg, G., et al. "Perioperative Myocardial Ischemia and Infarction: Identification by Continuous 12-lead Electrocardiogram with Online ST-Segment Monitoring," *Anesthesiology* 96(2):264-70, February 2002.

Mastering ACLS. Springhouse, Pa.: Springhouse Corp., 2002.

McAlister, F.A. "Atrial fibrillation, Shared Decision Making, and the Prevention of Stroke," *Stroke* 33(1):243-44, January 2002.

Wagner, G.S. *Marriott's Practical Electrocardiography,* 10th ed. Philadelphia: Lippincott Williams & Wilkins, 2001.

Index

---

i refers to an illustration; t refers to a table.

i refers to an illustration; t refers to a table.

i refers to an illustration; t refers to a table.

i refers to an illustration; t refers to a table.